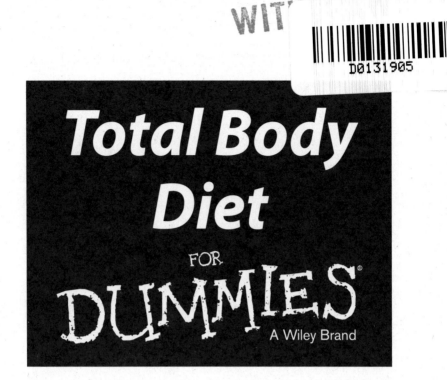

Total Body Diet

FOR

DUMMIES®

A Wiley Brand

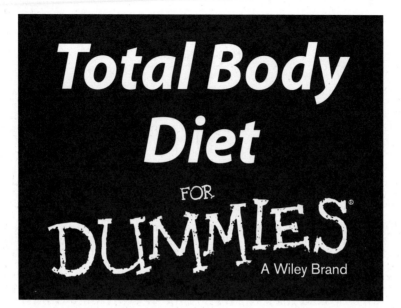

Total Body Diet

FOR DUMMIES®

A Wiley Brand

by Victoria Shanta Retelny

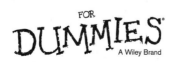

Total Body Diet For Dummies®

Published by: **John Wiley & Sons, Inc.,** 111 River Street, Hoboken, NJ 07030-5774, www.wiley.com

Copyright © 2016 by John Wiley & Sons, Inc., Hoboken, New Jersey

Published simultaneously in Canada

For general information on our other products and services, please contact our Customer Care Department within the U.S. at 877-762-2974, outside the U.S. at 317-572-3993, or fax 317-572-4002. For technical support, please visit www.wiley.com/techsupport.

Wiley publishes in a variety of print and electronic formats and by print-on-demand. Some material included with standard print versions of this book may not be included in e-books or in print-on-demand. If this book refers to media such as a CD or DVD that is not included in the version you purchased, you may download this material at http://booksupport.wiley.com. For more information about Wiley products, visit www.wiley.com.

Library of Congress Control Number: 2015960128

ISBN 978-1-119-11058-3 (pbk); ISBN 978-1-119-11054-5 (ebk); ISBN 978-1-119-11067-5 (ebk)

Manufactured in the United States of America

10 9 8 7 6 5 4 3 2 1

Contents at a Glance

Recipes at a Glance

Snacks and Desserts

Vegetarian

Table of Contents

Introduction

· ·

*W*ho doesn't want to be healthy, fit, and happy for life? With two out of three American adults being overweight or obese, weight loss is a common goal for many people to stave off health problems and poor quality of life. Many diets promise weight loss but only deliver temporary results — there's a need for a new approach. Losing weight isn't just about what you eat; it's also about your mental state, as well as your physical activity over the long term. It's your *total* body that counts!

In today's fast-paced society, instant gratification is highly sought after. So, people often overlook the slow steady changes that have proven to be the most effective for lasting results. Fad diets may prove effective over the short term, but they don't address the underlying reasons for weight gain, such as poor food choices, mindless eating, and/or lack of physical activity.

Ask yourself whether you're balanced in the main areas of your life: food, fitness, and mental health. From fueling your body right with optimal foods to embracing a regular physical activity routine to nurturing your psychological well-being with a mindful approach, *Total Body Diet For Dummies* offers a multidimensional, complete action plan to springboard you into a healthy lifestyle forever!

Through the tools, tips, and techniques in this book, you can develop a confidence around food to make healthy decisions anywhere, anytime. You'll feel truly empowered to break the reins of rigid diets and learn to choose from a bounty of nutritious foods that add color, texture, and taste that will fuel your body and mind.

About This Book

At first, adopting the Total Body Diet may seem like a daunting task, but this book makes it simple to tackle each of the principles gradually. As you embark on the journey of total body lifestyle changes, you'll understand what it means to get into a wellness mindset, as well as a physical one, too. You'll learn how to gauge your appetite, set boundaries with your food choices, and uncover your readiness to change. You'll see the value of different types of support — from working one-on-one with a registered dietitian nutritionist

(RDN) or another healthcare professional to garnering group support. Each chapter dives into something new, and you can read the book in any order that you choose!

The Total Body Diet gives you insight into what and how to eat to lose or maintain weight and lower your risk of chronic diseases like type-2 diabetes, cardiovascular disease, and cancer. It will also help you navigate the grocery story with more confidence to make healthier food choices. You'll discover options for getting physically active, as well as ways to incorporate move-ment into your everyday life.

Throughout the book, you'll see sidebars (text in gray boxes) — you can choose to read them or skip them. They give you a bit more in-depth informa-tion to give you a broader view of the topic area, but they aren't essential to your understanding of the topic at hand.

At the beginning of every recipe chapter, we include a list of the recipes in that chapter. Any vegetarian recipes are marked with a tomato icon (☺) so you can easily find them.

Within this book, you may note that some web addresses break across two lines of text. If you're reading this book in print and want to visit one of these web pages, simply key in the web address exactly as it's noted in the text, pretending as though the line break doesn't exist. If you're reading this as an e-book, you've got it easy — just click the web address to be taken directly to the web page.

Foolish Assumptions

As I was writing this book, I made some assumptions about you, the reader, so that I could home in on the focus of the book. Here are the assumptions I made about you:

- ✔ You want to live a long and healthy life and decrease your risk of chronic diseases.

- ✔ You want to connect with your mind and body in a way that is realistic to your lifestyle.

- ✔ You want to live your life mindfully with strategies to overcome mind-less eating.

- ✔ You want to reap the health benefits of physical activity and get tools, tips, and strategies for being more active.

Icons Used in This Book

Throughout this book, you'll see icons (small images in the margins) that are there to point out specific pieces of information. Here are the icons that I use along with a description of each:

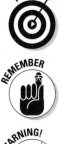

The Tip icon flags practical advice for furthering your knowledge and promoting total body wellness.

The information next to the Remember icon is so important that you should commit it to memory.

The Warning icon alerts you to something that may derail or sabotage your weight loss or healthy eating efforts.

When I go into greater detail on nutritional information than you need to understand the subject at hand, I mark those paragraphs with the Technical Stuff icon.

Beyond the Book

In addition to the material in the print or e-book you're reading right now, this product also comes with some access-anywhere goodies on the web:

- ✔ **Cheat Sheet** (www.dummies.com/cheatsheet/totalbodydiet)**:** The Cheat Sheet offers five simple strategies for weight loss, tips for balancing eating and activity, and guidance on eating right for energy.

- ✔ **Web Extras** (www.dummies.com/extras/totalbodydiet)**:** The Web Extras are free articles on subjects like debunking fad diets, herbs and spices for total body health, weight loss myths, and more.

Where to Go from Here

Now you're ready to dive into the Total Body Diet! I recommend starting with the first couple of chapters to get the gist of what total body wellness is all about, set your goals, and discover a new way of eating and living to improve your health and happiness. If you want some tasty recipes, skip to Part III, for meals, snacks, and healthy dessert ideas that your total body will benefit from and crave over and over again. Chapter 16 offers tech tools that can help you log your foods and beverages, track your sleep and activity, and create a more mindful lifestyle. Whatever your interest, take a peek at the table of contents or index to get the rundown and find what topic appeals to you now!

Part I

Getting Started with the Total Body Diet

getting started with

the total body diet

In this part . . .

- Tune into your total body wellness with mental and physical awareness.
- Set a new lifestyle to create lasting health changes.
- Know your hunger and fullness cues.
- Understand the power of sleep and ways to create a more restful environment.

Chapter 1

Talking Total Body Wellness

So, you want to embark on a lifestyle change that can promote health, well-being, and the quality of your life? The Total Body Diet offers a road map for a healthy mind and body by identifying nutrient-dense foods, ways to eat more mindfully, and keys to getting regular physical activity.

How can what you eat affect your total body health? Numerous studies have shown that a healthy pattern of eating has been linked to reduced risk of obesity, cardiovascular disease, high blood pressure, type 2 diabetes, some cancers, cognitive decline or dementia, and premature death, among other health benefits. Plus, research into physical activity shows benefits of improved flexibility, strength, mood, focus, and productivity.

Here are some key principles of the Total Body Diet:

✔ **Choose foods that are *minimally processed* (prepared without large amounts of added sugar, salt, and fat).** Minimize the additives you eat by checking labels and preparing foods at home with herbs and spices instead of a lot of salt, sugar, and fat.

✔ **Balance your daily eating plan with fruits, vegetables, whole grains, lean proteins (either animal or plant protein), and lowfat or fat-free dairy products.**

✔ **Drink water mainly.** Limit your consumption of beverages like regular soft drinks, alcoholic beverages, coffee, and tea.

✔ **Prepare meals and snacks at home.** You'll save calories with portion control and get less salt, added sugar, and solid fat.

✔ **Eat slowly and savor your food.** You'll reap the health benefits of mindful eating, which can help with the management of weight, type 2 diabetes, appetite, and cravings.

The Whole Picture of You

Before you can begin to make changes in your lifestyle, knowing where you are in your journey toward total body health and wellness is important. Ask yourself the following questions:

✔ Why do I want to make changes now? What is my goal?

✔ How ready am I to make this change? If it helps to quantify your readiness, rate yourself on a scale from 1 (not ready at all) to 5 (very ready).

✔ Am I willing to try new, healthier foods?

✔ Do I want to get more active or change my physical activity?

✔ Do I understand that change is a gradual process that takes time, patience, and daily action?

Think about your answers to these questions. If you're ready to change your lifestyle and create lasting changes, you're in the right place. It may take some time to get in the right frame of mind and find the motivation to power forward.

Tuning up your muscles

Regardless of your age or gender, your body and mind benefit from movement. According to the Physical Activity Guidelines for Americans, there is strong evidence that regular physical activity can help to decrease the risk of early death, cardiovascular disease, stroke, high blood pressure, weight gain, and depression among many other health benefits.

There are three key ways that physical activity benefits your total body wellness:

✔ **Overload:** Placing physical stress on your muscles, bones, heart, and lungs allows them to adapt to greater capacity and makes their function more efficient and stronger.

✔ **Progression:** Continually increasing your activity level, which overloads your body's systems, increases your fitness levels to enable you to keep doing more.

✔ **Specificity:** The type of activity you're doing benefits the specific body part that is doing the work (for example, aerobic activity works the cardiovascular system).

So what does this mean? If you aren't currently active, start slow and progress to a higher level slowly to build up your strength and *stamina* (the ability to sustain the activity for longer periods of time). For example, if you're new to activity, start with walking instead of running. When you're comfortable walking longer distances, start working in a little jogging at a time (a minute here or there, then two minutes, and so on). Creating small fitness goals to fine-tune your muscles gradually will lead to big results with persistence.

Getting into a wellness state of mind

The way you think about your health and wellness plays a role in the action you take toward living a healthier lifestyle. If you prioritize your health, you'll develop what I call a *wellness state of mind,* or a permanent healthy mindset. You'll think first and foremost about making the healthiest choice at the moment when it comes to food and physical activity. Instead of falling prey to unconscious eating and drinking, your new wellness mindset will help you become more focused on and conscious of your choices.

Wellness is not a one-size-fits-all proposition. Your wellness is unique to you, and it takes time to develop a wellness state of mind. It doesn't happen over-night. Be patient. Understand what you want and where you're starting from right now.

The Total Body Lifestyle

Embracing a healthy way of living for permanent, lasting changes is vital for creating improved health and wellness. The Total Body Diet is about adding beneficial foods, creating new behaviors, and fostering a sense of responsibil-ity to improve the quality of your life. Think about the value you're adding to your life by reaching your health goals — whether it be weight loss or main-tenance, reducing disease risk or managing current conditions, improved strength and flexibility, getting better sleep, or reducing stress.

It's beyond dieting — it's about living

This is not a typical diet plan, in which weight loss is the end all and be all. The Total Body Diet teaches you how to live with a greater awareness of how what *and* how you eat affects your mind and body for the better. It puts you on a path for greater understanding of how to navigate daily food choices, create more structure in your life, and eliminate the excuses that stand in your way to make significant health changes.

How do you get beyond the dieting mentality of eliminating certain foods? Many people struggle with the dieting mentality, so the foods they eliminate become taboo and may become the object of cravings as they're deemed "off-limits." This restrictive thinking makes food less enjoyable, too.

Balance is important. If you can, eat whole, minimally processed foods most of the time. Think about fueling your body with nutrient-dense food to keep your blood pressure, blood sugar, and waistline in check.

It's about changing your lifestyle! The Total Body Diet uses lifestyle as the first therapy to achieving wellness, health, and vitality for life. If you change your everyday behaviors and way of living, you'll see positive health outcomes above and beyond your dreams.

Making healthier food choices

Making healthier foods choices is challenging — even when you know what the better choice is. A 2014 Gallup poll asked Americans about their consumption habits and found that more than 90 percent of American adults *try* to include fruit and vegetables in their daily diets. But the Centers for Disease Control and Prevention's *State Indicator Report on Fruits and Vegetables* (2013) reveals that American adults eat fruit a mere 1.1 times per day and vegetables only about 1.6 times per day.

Let's face it — you're bombarded with a myriad of food choices every day. In fact, according to *Mindless Eating: Why We Eat More Than We Think,* by Brian Wansink, PhD, we make more than 200 decisions about food every day! Many of these choices are mindless — unless we tap into a more conscious, mindful way of eating.

A trip to the food court in your office building offers you a daunting number of food choices — from salads to soups to burgers and fries to pasta. What do you choose? Are you on automatic pilot and pick whatever sounds good at the moment? Or do you go there with a plan, with your sights set on making a healthy choice, which includes vegetables, fruits, lean protein, lowfat or fat-free dairy, and whole grains? It may sound simple, but without a plan, your healthy eating intentions can get easily sidetracked. So, what do you do? Set boundaries and create a healthier path.

Setting boundaries to create limitless possibilities

Every relationship in your life — including your relationship with food — thrives better with boundaries. If "anything goes" in a friendship, marriage, or relationship with a co-worker, that relationship can get out of control and unhealthy. Your needs may be ignored, taken advantage of, and minimized, if you don't clearly establish limits.

You may find it hard or easy to set boundaries, but whatever the case, knowing the importance of having limits with food is important to building a healthier relationship with food.

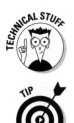

In the psychology world, *personal boundaries* are defined as the physical, emotional, and mental limits we establish to protect ourselves from being manipulated, used, or violated by others.

Here are seven simple steps to setting boundaries with food:

✔ **Eat nutrient-dense foods first,** *before* **highly processed, empty-calorie foods.** Color your plate with fruits and vegetables. Aim for at least 2 cups of fruit and 2½ cups of vegetables a day, as well as at least 3 servings of whole grains — *before* you eat refined grains with added sugar and solid fat, like cookies, crackers, and cake.

✔ **Go lean with protein.** Include plant proteins like beans and peas, tofu, nuts and seeds, seafood, skinless chicken and turkey breast, and loin cuts of beef or pork. Limit processed meats like bacon, salami, pepperoni, and prosciutto. Choose lowfat or fat-free dairy products — aim for 3 servings per day. A serving is 1 cup of milk, 1 cup of yogurt, 1½ ounces of hard cheese, or 2 ounces of soft cheese.

✔ **Keep calories light when it comes to beverages.** Avoid sugar-laden soft drinks, alcoholic beverages, and full-fat milk. Drink mostly water through the day!

✔ **Start your day with a balanced breakfast.** Aim to have a lean protein, whole grains, a piece of fruit or a vegetable, and one serving of lowfat or fat-free dairy.

✔ **Bring lunch and snacks with you to work or school to limit dining out in the afternoon.** You'll save money *and* calories.

✔ **Go grocery shopping with a list.** This way you have a plan going in and you'll minimize impulse purchases.

✔ **Don't eat chips, cookies, or crackers out of a box, bag, or carton.** Put a serving on a small plate or in a bowl and put the rest away.

Clueing into Your Appetite

Appetite awareness is a vital part of the Total Body Diet. Feeling hunger pangs and the satisfaction of a full stomach are key to healthy eating. Not only are you clueing into what your body needs, but you're also feeding your body's normal metabolic functions. The physical signs of hunger (a growling stomach, for example) keep you in tune with your appetite. In this section, I help you get intimate with your appetite. When you become attuned to your genuine appetite for food, you'll feel better about the food choices you're making on a daily basis.

Getting intimate with hunger and fullness

Do you know when you're hungry and when you're full? Identifying when your body really *needs* food is challenging, because for most of us, food is so readily available. We live in what I call a seductive eating environment, in which food temptations are everywhere. You may not be hungry, but the sights and aromas of nearby food may cause you to eat anyway. Although these are natural occurrences that are part of every day, you have to tune into them and realize that you don't have to eat chips just because they're on the table in front of you, and you don't have to grab a handful of candy out of your co-worker's candy jar just because it's sitting there. By tuning into your body's natural appetite gauges, you'll be more apt to pass up the extras and save room for nutrient-dense meals and snacks.

A great way to gain insight into hunger is to keep a journal. By jotting down your hunger (and fullness) before and after you eat, you can become more attuned to the appropriate times to eat and drink.

By definition, *hunger* is an uneasy sensation due to a lack of food, causing the stimulation of the sensory nerves of the stomach by the contraction and churning movement of the empty stomach. *Fullness* occurs at various levels, but it's having an appetite satisfied (not overly stuffed), especially for food or drink.

Knowing when to start and when to stop eating

Babies are born with an *innate* or natural ability to *self-regulate* — or an inner understanding of when to show signs of hunger and stop eating when full. Over time and with exposure to an abundant food environment, the ability to know when to start and when to stop eating becomes more difficult. How can you combat this in a world of oversized portions?

According to research in *Health Psychology* (2012) conducted by Brian Wansink, PhD, and his team at the Cornell Food and Brand Lab, if food had "stop signals," portion controlling food amounts would be a lot easier. In their study, 98 students were recruited from the University of Illinois and Pennsylvania State University. The students were given stacks of potato chips to munch on during a movie in class. Some had red dividers (or a tomato basil chip) placed within the chips (at every 7th chip and every 14th chip) and others just had yellow chips. The findings showed that the subjects who had dividers ate 50 percent less than the ones who didn't — about 250 calories less! Plus, the ones with dividers knew how many chips they ate — within

1 chip, whereas the others underestimated how much they had eaten by 12.6 chips!

What does this study reveal about knowing when to stop eating? Cues to stop eating are very effective. These cues can include things such as:

- ✔ Single-serve packages
- ✔ Snacks divided into serving-size bags
- ✔ Food placed on a plate and not eaten out of the bag, box, or carton
- ✔ Snacks that allow you to see how much you've eaten, like pistachios in shells

Understanding why you can't stop at one bite

You may relate to the following scenarios: You have one bite of chocolate cake, and it leads you to take another and another. Or you take one potato chip from the bag and that leads to eating half the bag. Or you have a spoonful of ice cream and keep going back for more. Why is it hard to stop at one bite, chip, or spoonful? It's not a mystery that foods high in added sugar, salt, and solid fat set us up to want to eat more. Sometimes the food is filling an emotional need brought on by feeling lonely or depressed. Even joyful and celebratory feelings bring on eating and overeating.

According to *The End of Overeating: Taking Control of the Insatiable American Appetite,* by David A. Kessler, MD, foods that are fatty, salty, and sugary tap receptors in the brain that release feel-good chemicals like dopamine, which make us want more of that food. Typically, those foods are high in calories, too — and they don't provide much in the way of nutrients.

These *trigger foods* can make you want to eat more. Not surprisingly, these are the foods that you want to limit on the Total Body Diet. Throughout this book, I give you helpful tools and strategies to limit these types of foods. Understanding what foods are trigger foods for you is life-changing and allows you to create a healthier relationship with food.

To identify your food triggers, write down which foods you cannot stop eating once you start. For example, write the following statement and fill in the blank:

> Once I start eating _____, I can't stop.

Multiple foods may be trigger foods for you.

Now that you've identified foods that are triggers to overeat, avoid keeping those foods in the house or at work. Set limits around these foods in order to reach your Total Body Diet goals.

The saying "Out of sight, out of mind" applies to food, especially foods that excite our taste buds and other senses. The first rule of thumb is not to have tempting foods in plain sight. If you have these foods around, you'll eat them. Buy single-serve portions of ice cream, or go out for a single scoop, instead of having a half-gallon container in your freezer. Ice cream will be more like a treat when you do have it — and you'll enjoy and savor it more, too!

Recharging with Rest

How does sleep foster total body wellness? Recent research shows that a well-rested body and mind are essential to good health. Just as eating well and getting regular physical activity are important to your health, sleeping seven to nine hours at night is a must for revitalizing your energy, thinking, and muscle repair and recovery. Sleep science, a relatively new field of research, reveals how sleep can affect overall quality of life.

Your body and mind work hard while you're awake. Sleep allows your major organs like your heart, lungs, brain, muscles, and stomach to slow down and literally recharge. According to the National Sleep Foundation (www.sleep.org), here are some of the ways different parts of your body benefit from sleep:

- ✔ **Brain:** Cerebral spinal fluid is pumped more quickly through the brain while you sleep, clearing away waste from brain cells, so your brain is clean and clear for the day ahead.

- ✔ **Heart:** Your blood pressure and heart rate slow during sleep, giving the heart a break overnight.

- ✔ **Lungs:** Breathing slows and becomes very regular during sleep, easing the load on your lungs overnight.

- ✔ **Muscles and joints:** Growth hormone is released to rebuild muscles and joints while you sleep.

- ✔ **Stomach:** Eating a balanced meal with a bit of carbohydrates (like whole-grain pasta, brown rice, or whole-wheat bread) along with protein-rich foods (like turkey or cheese) with some healthy fats (like avocado or olive oil) can keep your stomach satisfied overnight, which helps you sleep more soundly.

Melatonin is a hormone that is secreted during the nighttime hours that regulates your natural sleep-wake cycle and conveys day and night to your body. Melatonin is produced in the body with the help of an amino acid, tryptophan, which is found in high-protein foods like turkey, milk, and cheese. Certain foods naturally contain melatonin, such as tomatoes, walnuts, rice, barley, strawberries, olive oil, wine, beer, and milk. However, before you go out and get these foods to aid in better sleep, a study in *Food & Nutrition Research* points out that the health benefits of diet-driven melatonin boosts seem not to be the product of any single food or nutrients present in the diet. So these food are not sure-fire sleep-aids. Still, it can't hurt to get more nutrient-dense plant foods, as well as a few doses of lowfat dairy every day!

Recognizing the power of catnaps

You get drowsy in the afternoon and nod off for 20 minutes. Is that beneficial? Yes! Naps can recharge your brain, boost your energy, and make you more alert for the rest of the day. Many cultures plan for naps on a daily basis, but in the United States, the hustle and bustle of life gets in the way of regular naps. Sleep deprivation can lead to major health issues like weight gain, high blood sugar, high blood pressure, and mood disorders like depression.

Whether snoozing during the day is planned or spontaneous, brief catnaps of 10 to 20 minutes can be good for your health, according to sleep science experts. The value of an afternoon nap can mean the difference between performing well at work or not, or between being happy or sad.

Plan a short nap in your day, if you can. According to the journal *Sleep,* a brief respite of sleep — 10 minutes — appeared to be the best for improved alertness and brain power. Longer naps of 30 minutes or more create groggy, sluggish feelings afterward.

Relishing your bedtime routine

You've had a long day at work, at school, or with the kids, and you deserve a good night's sleep. Some of the best ways to ensure a good night's sleep is to have a regular routine at night. If you have an established routine, you'll be more apt to stick with it and get better shuteye, too.

Here are tricks and tips for getting a sound night's sleep:

- **Establish a regular sleep schedule.** Go to bed at the same time every night and wake up at the same time every morning.

- **Keep your bedroom temperature cool.** For most people, about 67 degrees is ideal for sleep.

✔ **Take a warm bath or shower before you go to bed.** As you cool down, the drop in body temperature will make you feel sleepy.

✔ **Make your bedroom soothing and tranquil.** Choose comfortable bedding, low lighting, and soothing music.

✔ **Make sure the bed is just for sleeping and sex.** Limit television watching or using your smartphone or computer in bed because the light from these devices stimulates your brain, making it harder to sleep.

Sleep hygiene is not the shower you take before bed — it's the habits you put in place before bed, such as avoiding bright lights in the bedroom, using ear plugs or a sound conditioner, listening to soothing music before bed, and positioning the clock away from direct view so that it doesn't distract you from getting to sleep. Practice good sleep hygiene, and your body will thank you for it.

Identifying the importance of a good night's sleep

Your lifestyle greatly affects your sleep quality and patterns. What you eat, what you drink, and how physically active you are play a big role in how well you rest. Here are some lifestyle changes that you can make in your Total Body Diet that can help you sleep better, too:

✔ **Avoid caffeinated foods and beverages at least four hours before bed.** Caffeine is a stimulant, and it can make it harder to fall asleep. Go for decaffeinated coffee, or have herbal tea, which is naturally caffeine-free. Skip the chocolate cake or brownie (or have less) — the caffeine may affect your shuteye.

✔ **Limit alcoholic beverages close to bedtime.** Alcohol may make you drowsy at first, but it may cause you to wake up during the night, especially the second half of the night, when you're in rapid eye movement (REM) sleep — the restorative, dream phase. The more you drink, the greater the disruptions, according to sleep experts. Limit your nightcap to one standard drink (12 ounces of beer, 5 ounces of wine, or 1½ ounces of liquor), if you want one, and have it at least a few hours before bed.

Alcohol is one of the most commonly used over-the-counter sleep aids, according to a review in the journal *Alcohol.* However, it does the contrary: It disrupts sleep, causing insomnia, daytime sleepiness, and snoring or *sleep apnea* (a start-stop breathing pattern during sleep), leading to many other health problems. If you're dependent on alcohol to fall asleep, this could be a red flag to stop or evaluate whether you have a drinking problem. Seek professional help from your healthcare provider or an addiction specialist.

✔ **Work out earlier in the day.** Taking an evening boxing class or lacing up your running shoes at dusk may be tempting, but it can leave you feeling wired and then you may find it hard to unwind and get to sleep. Swap this more intense exercise in the evening for more relaxing activities like *yoga nidra,* which is a conscious deep sleep. There are many yoga nidra workshops and free downloadable audios available online.

✔ **Eat lighter at night.** If you eat a large, high-calorie, fatty meal in the evening, you're bound to have a harder time getting to sleep and staying there — you may wake up with heartburn or may toss and turn due to a full stomach.

Here are some smaller meal ideas for the evening:

- A 3-ounce piece of grilled fish, 1 cup of broccoli, and ½ cup of cooked brown rice

- 1 cup of tofu stir-fried with 1 cup of mixed veggies and ½ cup of cooked brown rice

- 2 cups of mixed greens salad with a 3-ounce sliced baked chicken breast and ½ cup of cooked whole wheat couscous

- 2 slices (or 2 ounces) of turkey breast, ½ medium avocado, and 1 cup mixed greens in a 6-inch whole-grain wrap

For nighttime snacks, try the following:

- 1 cup of plain lowfat Greek yogurt with 1 tablespoon of ground flax-seed and a 1 teaspoon drizzle of honey

- A piece of whole-grain toast with 1 tablespoon of peanut butter and a handful of grapes

- ½ cup of cottage cheese spread on a large rice cake and 1 small apple

- Two slices of turkey breast rolled up with two thin slices of cucumber and ½ slice of provolone cheese in each slice

Chapter 2

What Is the Total Body Diet?

*E*veryone follows a *diet,* a way of eating that is part of everyday life. Some diets support a healthy life and allow us to be active, happy, and productive, while others are *fads,* or short-time fixes that typically restrict a certain food group (think low-carb diets) or are extreme (think very low-calorie diets) and are not sustainable over the long run. The Total Body Diet is not just a fleeting diet that makes short-term promises; it's a lifestyle that will not only give you vitality and freedom to make food choices, but also help you build a healthy relationship with food for life.

The Principles of the Total Body Diet

The tenets of the Total Body Diet are steeped in a tradition of a sound mind and body: life balance, self-confidence, and social support from friends and family. The Total Body Diet homes in on the importance of all these factors equally. If one area of life is not in sync, the rest will be out of whack.

Keep in mind the following principles of the Total Body Diet:

✔ Balance your diet with foods from all food groups (vegetables, fruits, whole grains, plant and animal sources of protein, and fat-free or lowfat dairy products) to sustain growth, energy, and well-being.

✔ Get active every day with enjoyable movement. Try walking, jogging, running, biking, hiking, swimming, stair climbing, Pilates, yoga, or tai chi.

✔ Make your mental health a priority by fostering a positive attitude. Your mind plays a large role in your health and your relationship to what and how you eat and drink.

Aim to follow these principles by balancing calories in with calories out as much as possible. Allow for flexibility, such as a small sweet indulgence or a low-key, less-active day to recharge your body and mind — you'll be more likely to stick with it and achieve total body wellness.

Moderation and balance as far as nourishment spans cultures and ages. The ancient Indian philosophy, particularly yoga, incorporates *mitahara,* or the habit of moderation with food and drink as part of a balanced diet.

Counting Calories without Forgetting about Quality

You don't want to go overboard on calories, but the Total Body Diet is about the quality of the calories you're consuming overall. You can easily reach your calorie quota for the day with foods and beverages that provide empty calories like candy, cookies, cheese puffs, and sugary drinks, but where's the quality in those calories? In this section, I get you focused on quality control when it comes to your calories.

Qualifying your calories

Food should be enjoyable and fun, but thoughtful eating and drinking is important to good health. *Qualifying* your calories by assessing their nutritional value is a good idea. An occasional cupcakes or doughnut is fine, but it doesn't qualify to be on your regular eating plan because it doesn't fuel your body well over the long run. Quality calories provide your body with *micronutrients* (vitamins and minerals), as well as *macronutrients* (carbohydrates, proteins, and fats). So, when you're eating and drinking, think about what's in your food.

A key way to qualify your calories is to inspect the Nutrition Facts label (shown in Figure 2-1). Important things to look at on the Nutrition Facts label include the following:

✔ **Serving size:** Look here to find out the suggested amount in one serving. It's the basis for all the nutrition information on the label. If you eat two servings, you have to double all the other numbers, too.

Nutrition Facts

Serving Size 1 cup (228g)
Servings Per Container about 2

Amount Per Serving

Calories 250   Calories from Fat 110

% Daily Value*

Total Fat 12g	**18%**
Saturated Fat 3g	**15%**
Trans Fat 3g	
Cholesterol 30mg	**10%**
Sodium 470mg	**20%**
Total Carbohydrate 31g	**10%**
Dietary Fiber 0g	**0%**
Sugars 5g	
Proteins 5g	
Vitamin A	4%
Vitamin C	2%
Calcium	20%
Iron	4%

* Percent Daily Values are based on a 2,000 calorie diet.
Your Daily Values may be higher or lower depending on
your calorie needs:

	Calories:	2,000	2,500
Total Fat	Less than	65g	80g
Saturated Fat	Less than	20g	25g
Cholesterol	Less than	300mg	300mg
Sodium	Less than	2,400mg	2,400mg
Total Carbohydrate		300g	375g
Dietary Fiber		25g	30g

Figure 2-1:
The Nutri-
tion Facts
label.

For educational purposes only. This label does not meet the labeling
requirements described in 21 CFR 101.9.

Source: U.S. Food and Drug Administration

✔ **Calories per serving:** When you know your serving size, you can figure out the total calories based on the number of servings you consumed. For example, if the serving size is 1 cup and you eat 2 cups, double the calories and the other nutrients on the label.

✔ **Nutrients to limit:** Check the label for total fat, trans fat, saturated fat, cholesterol, and sodium. You want to keep these at a minimum.

✔ **Nutrients to boost:** Aim for more dietary fiber, vitamins A and C, calcium, and iron.

If words resound better for you than numbers, check the ingredients on the package first. The first five ingredients reveal a lot! If you see sugar, salt, and unhealthy fat (such as partially hydrogenated vegetable oil) near the beginning of the ingredient list, that's a food you'll want to limit or avoid. Some ingredients — like sugar — are used more than once in a food product, in different forms. For example, you may see sucrose as the second ingredient and corn syrup and molasses elsewhere on the list — all three of those are sugar.

Getting better-for-you calories

I'm all about fostering quality on your plate, so let's talk about strategies to get better-for-you calories without too much effort. When eating well becomes a lifestyle, making food choices that benefit your total body will be second nature. You're creating a new habit. By practicing healthy eating every day, you'll actually train your brain to want better-for-you foods.

Research on habit-formation, shows that within ten weeks you can form a new habit if you simply repeat an action over and over again in the same context. What better context than eating and drinking, which you have to repeat at least three times a day?

One of the tools that can help you develop healthy eating habits is a food journal. Don't worry — it doesn't have to be as tedious as you think. You can create a simple journal on your computer, on a smartphone, or in a notebook by your desk or bedside. In order for it to be an effective tool, pick the same time every day to jot down what you consumed — it could be right after you eat or drink anything or before bed. What you want to record is everything you ate and drank, where you were when you consumed it, and how you feel about your choice. If you're not happy with the choice you made, write down an idea for a healthier choice you could've made instead.

That way, you'll train your brain to think of those healthier options the next time.

Research shows that people who have lost significant amounts of weight and kept it off for five years or more keep food journals regularly. Numerous mobile apps can help you with this task (see Chapter 16 for some recommendations). More than anything it cements healthy eating habits — and that's the ultimate goal, right?

Checking in with yourself

Be sure to check in with yourself to assess how you're doing throughout the day. The Total Body Diet is not a rigid diet where you have to eat the same foods every day or any one food group is off limits. Instead, it's a diet where quality foods and beverages count. How do you know if you're choosing a good-quality nourishment?

Ask yourself some questions before eating and drinking:

- ✔ Is this a healthy food or is it highly processed with little nutrition?
- ✔ Does it contain a lot of added sugar?
- ✔ Does it contain more than 20 percent of the Daily Value of sodium?
- ✔ Does it contain a lot more than 20 percent of the Daily Value of saturated fat?

If you answered yes to the first question, you're off to a great start with that food choice! Whole foods are typically less processed and more nutrient-dense.

Nutrients from food help keep your blood flowing smoothly, keep your brain synapses firing well, and maintain your good eyesight and organs functioning. No one food can do it all — it's the synergy of nutrients in good-quality, nutrient-dense foods that do your body good. So, it's important to determine if there are beneficial properties in the combination of your food choices. Aim for the majority of your foods to be in line with an overall healthy, nutrient-dense eating pattern.

Why do good-quality foods support total body wellness? They're packed with vital nutrients that have important health benefits (see Table 2-1).

Table 2-1	How Specific Nutrients Benefit Your Total Body
Nutrient	*Benefit*
Protein	Maintains and builds your muscle mass.
Dietary fiber	May help reduce blood cholesterol levels; is important for proper bowel function; may reduce constipation.
Calcium	Keeps bones strong and healthy.
Vitamin D	Helps strengthen bones.
Vitamin C	Helps to maintain collagen in skin and defend cells from free radicals.
Vitamin A	Important for eye health and the immune system.
B vitamins	Eight vitamins (thiamin, riboflavin, niacin, pantothenic acid, B6, biotin, folic acid, and B12) that are critical for numerous functions in your body, including obtaining energy from the foods you eat.
Potassium	Helps control blood pressure by regulating fluid in and between cells.
Fats	Unsaturated fats like omega-3 fatty acids (DHA and EPA) are beneficial for cardiovascular health and inflammation.

Let's Get Physical!

Activity plays a large role in maintaining your total body wellness. If you're sedentary, research shows that your risk of chronic diseases like cancer, heart disease, and obesity goes up. So, reducing the amount of time you sit every day is vital.

Think about ways to reduce your sitting time. Can you work at a standing desk or get up more and move during the day?

Moving improves health, and there's oodles of research to prove it! Global initiatives like the Healthy Eating Activity and Lifestyle (HEAL) program in Australia recruited 2,827 participants to complete an hour of physical activity once a week followed by an hour of lifestyle education for eight weeks. The results were positive, with participants reducing total body mass, waist circumference, and blood pressure. The Women's Health Initiative, a 15-year study of women ages 50 to 79, revealed that less time spent sitting reduced the risk of death among the more than 92,000 participants over the course of the study.

Knowing how much movement you need

The Physical Activity Guidelines for Americans recommends that adults move more — to the tune of at least 150 minutes of moderate-intensity physical activity per week. How you schedule your activity is up to you. You may choose to do 30 minutes five times per week or 50 minutes three times per week — but spreading it out over the course of the week is preferable. With our increasingly sedentary lifestyle, it's vital to make a conscious effort to move daily. Even ten-minute increments throughout the day will work wonders!

If you don't do any regular activity now, start slowly and increase the amount and intensity gradually.

There are two types of activity, according to the Physical Activity Guidelines for Americans:

- ✔ **Baseline or lifestyle activity:** Light-intensity activity of daily life like standing, walking slowly, and lifting lightweight objects. You're considered inactive if this is all you do.

- ✔ **Health-enhancing physical activity:** Goes over and above the basic activities of daily living and can improve your health.

You can make activity fun and do what you enjoy! You might enjoy brisk walking, running, jumping rope, cycling, dancing, lifting weights, climbing, swimming, or yoga.

Reducing the time you spend on your keister

Although, it's a good practice to sit when you eat (because you'll eat more slowly and mindfully), how can you avoid sinking into your easy chair in the evening or collapsing on the couch when you get home? Now, I'm not suggesting that you *never* sit down, but finding pleasure from other activities is a smart, healthy idea.

A good way to limit your sitting time is to try never to sit more than 90 minutes at one time. Here are some tips for sprinkling physical activity in throughout your day:

- ✔ Walk or bike to and from school or work or to and from the train or bus.

- ✔ Walk to grab lunch or sneak in a 30-minute lunchtime workout at your local gym. Your workplace may even have a small gym onsite — if the weather is bad, you could walk on the treadmill for 30 minutes before you eat.

✔ Stretch at your desk or when you get home. Instead of sitting in front of the TV, stretch for 10 to 15 minutes while you watch your favorite show.

✔ Park your car farther away from the store to get a longer walk.

✔ Walk your dog when you get home or talk a walk after dinner, if you don't have a pet.

✔ Walk to a co-worker's desk instead of sending an email.

✔ Take the stairs instead of the elevator.

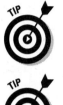

If you sit a lot at work and your job allows, set a timer for every 20 to 30 minutes. When the timer rings, get up and stretch or walk around the office. That'll get the blood flowing to your organs, arms, and legs.

See if you can get a variable desk that lowers when you want to sit a bit and raises so you can stand up and work, too. Check out one option at www.varidesk.com.

Stretching your way to good health

Strength and flexibility are a big part of health. Stretching can improve athletic performance, as well as decrease risk of injuries.

Before your stretch, consult with your healthcare provider or physical therapist, particularly if you have an injury. Although stretching is a key part of a healthy lifestyle, you can injure yourself or aggravate an existing injury if you don't know what you're doing.

Here are some tips for stretching well:

✔ **Stretch when warm.** Don't stretch as soon as you wake up or when your muscles are cold. Stretch after you're warmed up by either walking, lightly jogging, or biking to get blood pumping in your arms and legs.

✔ **Avoid pain.** Forget that old adage "No pain, no gain." You never want to push the stretch to the point of pain.

✔ **Strive for symmetry with your stretches.** Your goal is equal flexibility on each side.

✔ **Smooth out your stretches.** Avoid bouncing — it can cause a muscle injury.

✔ **Time your stretches.** Hold each stretch for 30 to 60 seconds, but don't hold your breath. Breathe in and out normally.

✔ **Schedule your stretches.** To make stretching part of your routine, aim for at least two to three times per week. It's great to cool down with stretching, too.

✔ **Stretch to your sport.** For example, runners or basketball players should focus on hamstrings; tennis players should focus on arms, shoulders, and quadriceps.

Getting Psyched: Keeping in Mind Your Mental Health

Taking the plunge into the Total Body Diet isn't a solo process. Getting social support from family and friends, as well as professionals, can be a tremendous help.

Think about these folks as being part of your Total Body Diet team. Assembling an effective team around you can help in many ways. There is nothing like having other people rooting for you when you're starting a new behavior change program. Getting support from a team is not a new concept — organizations and institutions all over the world use an interdisciplinary approach to healthy behavior change, especially when it comes to healthful eating, weight loss, or weight maintenance.

Your team may consist of a whole host of professionals, including the following:

✔ Registered dietitian nutritionists

✔ Nurses and nurse practitioners

✔ Pharmacists

✔ Physicians

✔ Physician assistants

✔ Physical therapists

✔ Psychologists

✔ Social workers

You may not choose to work with all these people at once, but knowing the range of help available allows you to reach out for appropriate support when necessary. Also, you may not be working one-on-one with every one of these folks — for example, a nutritionist may lead a support group you can join.

The benefits of cognitive behavioral therapy

Cognitive behavioral therapy (CBT) is short-term therapy that focuses on the relationship between thoughts, feelings, and behaviors in the present and strategies to problem-solve. It's administered by a clinical psychologist or trained, licensed therapist. The professional and patient work actively together to build skills, set goals, and structure therapy sessions.

CBT has proven to be successful for weight loss. In fact, it's one of the most popular therapies for weight management. Recent research in the *Journal of Clinical Psychology* shows that overweight people who are struggling with weight loss prefer CBT to other therapies. It's comprehensive and practical. Plus, CBT allows people to build self-care skills and healthy goals and see concrete results.

Family members should also be on your team. They can be your cheerleaders for personal change! The Total Body Diet approach encourages the whole family to get onboard with lifestyle changes.

Support begins in the home. Talk with your spouse, kids, siblings, and/or parents to make them aware that you're transforming your eating and lifestyle for the better. Ask them for support!

Ready, Set, Go! A Self-Assessment

Change is the only constant in life, so why do we find it so difficult to make lifestyle changes? Maybe because we're creatures of habit. If you surrender to the fact that change is a fluid, dynamic force in your life, change will come more easily and be more rewarding.

Here are five key ways to embrace the challenge of change every day:

- ✔ **Bite off small pieces.** When you've identified an area that you want to change, take small steps to address it every day. Slowly but surely you'll see big results unfold in your life.

- ✔ **View change in a new way.** Instead of viewing change as challenging, view it as an opportunity to learn and grow. You'll be more apt to move forward if you see this as a journey filled with learning.

- ✔ **Foster a sense of gratitude for the change.** Instead of denying that you need to change a behavior or area of your life, be grateful for this call to action ahead. It's an opportunity for self-improvement.

- ✔ **Help others make changes.** When you've identified and made small changes in your life, helping others in your community to make changes is a great way to cement changes in your own life.

✔ **Practice, practice, practice.** Focus less on perfection and more on progress. Even if you falter, the act of practicing will allow you to get back on track right away.

The assessment in Table 2-2 identifies areas where change is needed the most. Using a scale of 1 to 10 (where 1 is rarely and 10 is always), rate your effort.

Table 2-2	Total Body Assessment
Behavior	*Rating*
Nourishment	
You make food choices based on the quality of the food available.	
You use portion control with your meals and snacks.	
You get at least 2½ cups of vegetables per day.	
You get at least 2 cups of fruits per day.	
You eat at least half of your grains from whole-grain sources.	
You choose lean protein sources (such as skinless poultry, seafood, loin cuts of beef or pork, and tofu).	
You eat legumes weekly.	
You drink at least 1 cup per day of lowfat or fat-free milk or calcium-fortified soymilk.	
You eat at least 1 cup of lowfat or fat-free yogurt daily.	
You eat no more than 1½ ounces of lowfat or reduced-fat cheese daily.	
You plan your grocery visits with a list.	
You try not to skip meals.	
You bring lunch and snacks with you.	
You drink water throughout the day.	
You limit alcoholic beverages (no more than one drink per day for women and two drinks per day for men).	
You feel good and have a sense of gratitude for your food and choices.	
Subtotal	
Movement	
You are physically active most days of every week.	
You do aerobic activity (such as spinning, running, speed walking, or swimming).	

(continued)

Table 2-2 *(continued)*

Behavior	Rating
Movement	
You do muscle-strengthening activities (such as free weights, weight machines, yoga, or Pilates).	
You enjoy the physical activities you do.	
You have realistic, achievable goals.	
You have an exercise buddy.	
You are mindful of moving during the day (for example, standing at work, walking to or from work or school, and parking farther away).	
You exercise your mind by reading and doing crossword puzzles or games (such as Sudoku).	
Subtotal	
Social Engagement	
You go out with your spouse or partner on a regular basis.	
You make plans with friend(s) at least once a week.	
You engage in other social group activities at least twice a month.	
You foster new relationships or friendships.	
You connect with friends on a regular basis.	
You go on at least one vacation per year.	
Subtotal	
Total	

Now tally up your score for each section, and your total. The higher the total score (the maximum you can score is 300), the more attuned you are to your physical and mental needs. To find areas for focus, circle the questions that had a lower score. These are the ones that need more attention. You can also look at the subtotals for each of the three sections — maybe you scored high on social engagement, but you're falling short on movement and nourishment. If so, keep up the great work socially, but focus your efforts on what you eat and how much you move.

Now that you know where you need to make changes, sit with your assessment for a few minutes. Take a few deep breaths. Think about which areas you want to tackle first. When you have a couple of ideas that resonate with you, begin embarking on your change adventure!

Chapter 3

Managing Your Waistline and Beyond

*Y*our blood says a lot about you and your health. From your food choices to physical activity to your genetic makeup, there's no hiding it from your blood. That's why your doctor should test your blood every year. Blood tests show if your organs are functioning in tip-top shape and if different substances in your blood fall within a healthy range. Blood test ranges depend on a number of variables, like age, gender, race, and other factors (such as stress, pregnancy, and hormone cycles).

Every time you get a blood test, request a copy and discuss the results with your healthcare provider. From blood cell counts to kidney function to liver enzymes, deciphering your report can be difficult. Unless you know what the numbers mean, it may seem like a foreign language to you.

In this chapter, I home in on the quality of what's in your blood. You find out what your numbers mean to your overall health. I give you the scoop on the big health indicators — cholesterol (both the good and bad types), blood sugar, and blood pressure. Finally, I focus on how changes in eating, exercise, and overall lifestyle can help reduce your disease risk.

Health in Numbers

The great thing about your first blood test is that it establishes a baseline from which you can go up, down, or stay the same. You can use your blood tests from year to year as an assessment tool to determine if you're where you want to be and what, if any, action plan you're going to put in place.

A number of different blood tests look at different things in the blood. A comprehensive metabolic panel looks at blood glucose (sugar), calcium, electrolytes (sodium, potassium, bicarbonate, and chloride), protein levels, as well as kidney and liver function. A complete blood count (CBC) determines the volume of red and white blood cells and platelets, as well as iron stores with hemoglobin and hematocrit levels. A lipoprotein panel assesses cardiovascular disease risk by homing in on lipids like total cholesterol, low-density lipoproteins (LDL), high-density lipoproteins (HDL), and triglycerides.

Depending on the type of blood test, there will be a different dietary protocol in place. Always consult with your healthcare provider beforehand to find out what you can (and can't) eat. The following guidelines usually apply before blood tests, but consult with your healthcare provider to confirm the pre-blood test protocol:

- ✔ Fast (do not eat any food) 8 to 12 hours prior to the blood test.

- ✔ Hydrate well with water.

- ✔ Do not drink alcohol.

- ✔ If taking medications or supplements (including vitamins), ask your healthcare provider whether you can take them prior to a blood test.

Your blood is dynamic matter — it's always changing — so your numbers can change over time. That means if your test results aren't where you want them to be, you can make lifestyle changes that change your test results for the better! Knowing your numbers can help you take action toward getting your numbers where you need them to be.

Clearing Up Cholesterol Confusion

One of the biggest blood indicators of heart health is *cholesterol,* the waxy substance made naturally in your liver that may block arteries, if overproduced, overconsumed, or not excreted from the body properly. The confusion with cholesterol is that there are different types of it — some cholesterol particles (depending on their size) do your body good and others cause harm, if left to their own devices.

Differentiating the types of cholesterol

Cholesterol gets a bad rap as far as heart health goes, but did you know that some types of cholesterol actually protect the heart? The good type is called high-density lipoproteins (HDL). As its name implies, HDL is denser, so it actually sweeps through the arteries and clears away the less-dense particles. The low-density lipoproteins (LDL) can actually stick to walls of the arteries causing blockages, or *atherosclerosis.* The goal is to get the good stuff up and the bad stuff down.

Along with cholesterol other blood *lipids* (fats) called *triglycerides* are important. You want to keep triglycerides in a healthy range to prevent heart disease. If your triglycerides are high, cut back on refined carbohydrates like cookies, candies, cake, crackers, white bread, and alcohol. Replacing refined carbohydrates with polyunsaturated fats like omega-3 fatty acids from fatty fish like salmon, tuna, and trout can help, too.

Healthy cholesterol numbers look like this:

Total cholesterol: Less than 200 mg/dL

HDL: 60 mg/dL or greater

LDL: Less than 130 mg/dL or less than 100 mg/dL if you have cardiovascular disease

Triglycerides: Less than 150 mg/dL

Individual labs may have different ranges that they consider healthy. If you have a question about your cholesterol results, consult your healthcare provider.

Is it really bad to eat cholesterol?

The cholesterol you eat — also called *dietary cholesterol* — is found only in animal-based foods, and it's no longer on the taboo list. The latest Dietary Guidelines for Americans, which are a scientific road map for nutrition education and guidance, shows that the research is lacking on the relationship between eating cholesterol-laden foods (say, egg yolks and shellfish) and a lot of cholesterol circulating in your bloodstream causing blocked arteries. Of course, it's smart to practice moderation with all foods.

All plant foods are naturally cholesterol-free and can help improve cholesterol numbers. So eat them to your heart's content (no pun intended!).

Focusing on food

Some foods can help lower the "bad" cholesterol (LDL) and/or raise the "good" (HDL) cholesterol. By adding the beneficial, cholesterol-lowering foods to your diet, you can make strides in decreasing your risk for heart disease.

The right type of fat — the unsaturated type — can be beneficial for raising "good" (HDL) cholesterol, as well as lowering the bad cholesterol. There are two types of unsaturated fats: monounsaturated and polyunsaturated fats. A combination of these fats exists in many foods, but some foods have higher levels of one type. Foods with unsaturated fats can improve your ratio of LDL to HDL. These include monounsaturated fats like the following:

- Canola oil, olive oil, peanut oil, high oleic safflower oil
- Pistachios, almonds, pecans, and peanuts
- Almond butter and peanut butter
- Avocadoes

Polyunsaturated fats like the following also help the LDL-to-HDL ratio:

- Salmon, halibut, tuna, mackerel, herring, and trout
- Walnuts
- Flaxseeds, chia seeds, and hemp seeds
- Soybeans and tofu
- Soybean oil

Eating plant foods like fruits, vegetables, legumes, whole grains, and nontropical vegetable oils may help lower LDL and total cholesterol because they contain naturally occurring compounds called *plant stanols* and *plant sterols.*

Research has shown that consuming 2g to 3g of plant sterols per day may lower total cholesterol by 7 percent to 11 percent and LDL levels by 7 percent to 15 percent as they block the absorption of cholesterol in the small intestine. Foods fortified with plant sterols, such as spreads, yogurts, and orange juice, have shown promise for people at risk for cardiovascular disease with elevated LDL.

When choosing spreads, be sure to check labels for trans fats or partially hydrogenated vegetable oil because they pose a risk for cardiovascular disease. Also, beware: You need two 8-ounce glasses of fortified orange juice per day to reach the therapeutic dosage of plant sterols — and that's a lot of excess calories!

Beside just your dietary choices, lifestyle changes — such as quitting smoking, losing weight, and getting regular physical activity — can help bring cholesterol levels down and reduce your risk of heart disease.

Becoming Blood Sugar Savvy

Your blood *glucose* (sugar) levels reveal a lot about your health. With 21 million people in the United States diagnosed with diabetes and 8.1 million walking around undiagnosed, it's important that you know your blood sugar trends. If your blood glucose levels are high often (as with prediabetes or full-blown diabetes), this can wreak havoc on many organs in your body — your heart, eyes, brain, and nerves can all be affected. The longer your blood sugar stays elevated, the more damage may be done. You don't want your blood sugar diving too low either. *Hypoglycemia* (low blood sugar) can be a precursor to diabetes.

If you feel nausea, sluggish, irritable, confused, or mentally foggy, your blood sugar may be too high or low. Still, blood sugar control is more than just paying attention to how you feel throughout the day because you may not feel anything different. Testing your blood sugar at regular times throughout the day can give you insights into how your blood sugar is trending.

If you don't have diabetes, you're probably not testing your blood sugar yourself. Your doctor should test it at your yearly physical. You'll likely have to fast for at least eight hours before your blood is drawn. Normal fasting blood glucose is between 70 and 99 mg/dL. If your fasting blood glucose is between 100 and 125, you have prediabetes. And if your fasting blood glucose is 126 or above, you have full-blown diabetes.

On the other hand, if your blood sugar levels are too low — less than 70 mg/dL — you have hypoglycemia, which is caused by a number of things, including the following:

✔ Not eating for a long time

✔ Your *pancreas,* the organ that produces insulin, producing more than needed

✔ Taking too much insulin or certain medications

The goal is to keep your blood sugar in the healthy range for the long haul. And you can do that with diet and exercise.

Controlling blood sugar

Blood sugar responds well to rules and regulations. A regular schedule of eating, drinking, and exercise does your blood sugar good. When your schedule is out of whack, chances are, your blood sugar is, too!

Here are the Total Body Diet rules for blood sugar control:

- ✔ **Wake up and eat.** Eat within one to two hours of waking up in the morning.
- ✔ **Combine food groups.** Have protein-rich foods with complex carbohydrates and healthful fats with meals and snacks.
- ✔ **Eat often.** Space your meals and snacks regularly through the day to stabilize blood sugar.
- ✔ **Move more.** Get daily physical activity.

The combination of foods you choose to eat every day affects your blood sugar. When planning your meals and snacks, opt for whole, less processed foods first.

Watching the added sugar

Sugar occurs naturally in foods — for example, lactose is found in milk and yogurt, and fructose is found in fruit — and it is also added to food products in many different forms. Examine the Nutrition Facts label to determine what nutrients the food provides for your body. Food products with added sugars can contain too much sugar and typically don't have as much to offer in the way of nutrients.

Whichever form sugar comes from, your body needs to get that glucose into your cells with the help of insulin. Your pancreas releases insulin in response to the amount of glucose (sugar) in your blood to facilitate it getting into your cells to be used as energy. However, if there is more fiber, protein, or fat in the food, it will thwart the blood sugar spike and give your pancreas a break from having to kick out too much insulin. So, eating more whole foods — even if they contain natural sugar — is better than eating food products with a lot of added sugar in them.

Sugar has many substitutes. If you choose to eat foods or beverages sweetened with artificial sweeteners, such as extracts from stevia (Truvia or Purvia), monkfruit (Nectresse), sucralose (Splenda), or aspartame (Equal), assess the Nutrition Facts Panel. Just because the sweeteners are low or no calorie, doesn't mean the products are. Err on the side of less is more when it comes to sugar substitutes.

Beverage watch

When you think about what to drink for your total body health, think water. Not only does water hydrate your body, but it fills you up with zero calories and helps with appetite control, too. Research shows that drinking water before a meal results in less food consumed at the meal, because water takes the hunger edge off. Also, if you eat foods with more water like fruits and vegetables, you'll fill up faster on fewer calories. And that's a bonus!

Monitor calories in other beverages, such as gourmet coffees, juices, alcohol, and enhanced water and sports drinks. The calories can add up fast! As you're jotting down what you eat, include beverages, too — it's eye-opening to see where extra calories and added sugars are coming in!

According to a recent report by the Centers for Disease Control, 63 percent of American adults drink sugar-sweetened beverages every day. They get 9 percent of total calories, or 203 calories per day, from sugary beverages. If you're among those who like sugar-sweetened beverages, consider strategies to cut back:

- If you crave carbonation, drink sparkling water with a twist of lemon or lime.

- Add a splash of juice to water to get the flavor without excess calories.

- Try drinking milk (cow's milk, almond milk, hazelnut milk, coconut milk, or hemp milk) instead.

A teaspoon of table sugar is 15 calories. The typical American eats 16 percent of his daily calories from *added sugars* or sugars added during food production. Think about it — do you check food labels for sugars? The good news is, soon you'll be able to sleuth out sugars added during processing! The Food and Drug Administration (FDA) has proposed changes to the Nutrition Facts label to specify not just sugars, but added sugars, too!

Keeping Your Blood Pressure in Check

Blood pressure is a powerful player in heart health. One in three people has *high blood pressure* or a blood pressure reading of 140/90 or higher. At any given time your blood pressure can boil up due to stress, intense activity, or even lack of sleep.

Normal blood pressure is less than 120/80. You may have lower blood pressure naturally. That's not unhealthy as long as there are no underlying symptoms like light-headedness, fatigue, excessive thirst, nausea, blurred vision, or depression.

Low and high blood pressure readings are a red flag to talk with your health-care provider. In either case, real food and lifestyle changes can help get it under control.

Befriending potassium-rich foods

Do you ever think about getting enough potassium? Probably not. One of the major functions of this mineral is to keep blood pressure in check. Potassium works opposite to sodium (salt) — it helps to maintain the delicate fluid balance by allowing your kidneys to release water from the bloodstream, reversing sodium's grip on your body's water stores.

Natural, food sources of potassium are best. You need 4,700 mg per day, unless your kidneys are not functioning properly. In that case, consult with your healthcare provider.

Unless prescribed by your doctor, avoid potassium supplements — they can cause dangerous symptoms like irregular heart rhythm, low blood pressure, and even death.

Try these potassium all-stars:

- ✔ **Vegetables:** Potatoes (with skin), sweet potatoes (with skin), spinach, zucchini, tomato, kale

- ✔ **Fruits:** Avocado, banana, apricot, cantaloupe, orange

- ✔ **Nuts, seeds, and legumes:** Soybeans, lentils, white beans, split almonds, pistachios, sunflower seeds, peanuts

- ✔ **Dairy products:** Milk, yogurt

- ✔ **Meat and fish:** Lean cuts of beef and pork, salmon, halibut, tuna

Limiting high-sodium foods

Sodium occurs in many foods naturally, and it's also added to foods for a variety of reasons — from flavor enhancement to helping baked goods to rise to preserving and tenderizing meat and fish. However, too much sodium puts you at risk for a heart attack or stroke.

You can cut your sodium easily by doing the following:

- ✔ **Limiting highly processed foods:** Eating fresh whole foods cuts back on salt significantly. When choosing minimally processed foods, be sure to check the Nutrition Facts label for sodium. Less than 5 percent of the Daily Value is low; greater than 20 percent of the Daily Value is high. A low-sodium food contains 140 mg or less of sodium per serving.

✔ **Dining out less:** When you prepare your meals and snacks at home, you not only have greater control over the amount of sodium you eat, but also cut back on calories (and money!).

✔ **Using herbs and spices to flavor food:** Instead of reaching for the salt shaker, use herbs and spices. If you're using an herb or spice rub or blend, check the label because it may contain salt.

Herbs and spices are a better alternative to decreasing salt than salt substitutes, which typically contain a lot of potassium chloride, which can be dangerous if you have a kidney problem or are on medication for heart, kidneys, or liver.

✔ **Sticking with unsalted butter, nuts, and seeds.**

✔ **Purchasing low-sodium versions of foods:** In low-sodium versions, the salt is cut by at least 50 percent from the original version. You can find low-sodium soy sauce, prepared meats, fish, cheeses, soups, cottage cheese, canned vegetables, and beans.

Putting a lock on stress and anxiety

Chronic stress and anxiety can cause your blood pressure to soar and lead to eventual heart problems. The link between the mind-body connection and cardiovascular disease is a proven phenomenon and one that deserves attention. One in five patients with coronary artery disease or heart failure is depressed — that's three times greater than the prevalence of depression in the greater population, according to a 2015 review in the *American Journal of Hypertension.* Several large and small studies conducted over the last five years show that psychological disorders, such as depression, stress/post-traumatic stress disorder, and anxiety are connected to cardiovascular disease.

So what can you do? I created the RELAX method for Total Body Dieters. Here it is:

✔ **R**elate to your mental state. In other words, identify how you're feeling — whether it's stressed, anxious, or depressed.

✔ **E**valuate your feelings regularly and take a step back to look at them.

✔ **L**augh out loud every day to alleviate heavy feelings.

✔ **A**sk for help from a professional.

✔ **X** out days on your calendar or items on your list to show progress that can affect your heart health.

Clamping down on alcohol

Over time, excessive drinking (more than 3 drinks on any day or 7 drinks per week for women and more than 4 drinks on any day or 14 drinks per week for men) can cause blood pressure to rise, as well as other health problems. With alcohol, moderation is key. A glass of red wine a day may benefit heart health, but more than that can disrupt your sleep patterns, slow you down, and worsen depression, stress, and anxiety.

What does one drink look like? That's 5 ounces of wine, 12 ounces of beer, or 1½ ounces of liquor.

If you drink alcohol, pair it with food. Drinking on an empty stomach can cause blood sugar to fall and excessive overeating later. Drink slowly, dilute wine or liquor with sparkling water, and always put a limit of one drink per day for women and two drinks per day for men. Your heart, liver, and waistline will all thank you later!

Keeping Tabs on Your Waistline

Your waistline reveals a lot about your health. Belly fat plays an important role in cardiovascular disease, type 2 diabetes, and cancer, so you want to find ways to keep your waistline in a healthy range for you.

Making friends with your tape measure

Your bathroom scale doesn't tell you if you've gained fat or muscle (unless you have a special scale that detects body fat percentage). How your clothes fit reveals a lot. Using your clothes as a waistline gauge is wise, but a tape measure is the best possible tool.

Follow these steps to measure your waist circumference accurately:

1. **Stand straight upright, and place the end of the tape measure just above your hip bone.**

2. **Slowly wrap it around your waist until it meets up with the other end (level with your belly button), as shown in Figure 3-1.**

3. **Exhale and then look down at the number.**

   That's your waist circumference. Write it down with the measurement date for future reference.

Figure 3-1:
Measuring
your waist
circumfer-
ence.

A healthy waistline measures less than 35 inches for non-pregnant women and less than 40 inches for men.

You can also calculate your *waist-to-hip ratio* (the size of your hips compared to the size of your waist) to determine if you're carrying a high percentage of body weight in your abdomen. In a similar fashion to measuring your waistline, you can use a tape measure to measure the circumference of your waist-to-hip ratio. To do this, look in the mirror and determine the widest part of your buttocks and wrap the tape measure from that point around your hips to find the circumference of your hips and buttocks. Then using your hip measurement, divide your waist circumference by your hip measurement and that's your waist-to-hip ratio. It's that easy!

There are risks for disease states associated with a high waist-to-hip ratio. See Table 3-1 to determine your risk level:

Table 3-1	Waist-to-Hip Ratio and Risk	
Male Waist-to-Hip Ratio	*Female Waist-to-Hip Ratio*	*Health Risk*
0.95 or below	0.80 or below	Low
0.96 to 1	0.81 to 0.85	Moderate
1.0+	0.85+	High

Another measure of risk for disease is *body mass index* (BMI), which is mea-sure of your height-to-weight ratio. You can calculate yours at www.nhlbi. nih.gov.

The best part about keeping tabs on your waist circumference is that it can keep you honest with how you've been eating and drinking. Plus, if you need to get more active or change up your exercise routine the inches don't lie.

When planning your regular waistline check-ins, strategize the timing. Whether you're a man or a woman, the best bet is to take your measure-ment in the morning, right after waking. Also, you want to measure the day after a typical day — the Monday after a weeklong cruise or the day after Thanksgiving are not the best times to measure your waist! Aim to measure your waistline every month. Pick the same day of the month, such as the first of the month. (Women should avoid measuring right before or during their menstrual cycles, because bloating tends to occur and the measurement may not be accurate.)

Deciphering the story your waistline is revealing

A svelte, trim waistline is not only healthy and makes you feel good in your body, but it reveals a lot from a metabolic standpoint. The medical com-munity has examined belly fat for decades, and the findings have revealed that *abdominal adiposity* (fat around the midsection) can be dangerous to your health.

Regardless of your age, carrying too much belly fat can lead to a cluster of symptoms called *metabolic syndrome*. Five factors are important when it comes to metabolic syndrome:

- ✔ High fasting blood glucose
- ✔ High triglycerides
- ✔ Low HDL cholesterol,
- ✔ High blood pressure
- ✔ A large waistline

If you have three of these five factors, you have metabolic syndrome. And that increases your risk for heart disease, stroke, and diabetes.

The middle bulge is not inevitable

You may think that history repeats when it comes to your body size and shape, but that's not necessarily true — you can influence your own health history! Even if your family members have tended to carry extra weight, you can produce change in your own life.

Hormones can play a role in the belly bulge. For young women with *polycystic ovarian syndrome* (PCOS), a hormonal disorder characterized by cysts around the outer edge of one or both ovaries, there is a tendency to gain weight around the middle. Likewise, hormonal fluctuations during the onset of perimenopause and menopause, when estrogen production wanes and eventually stops, can lead to weight gain around the waist; fat is no longer stored around the hips for reproductive purposes but moves up toward the abdomen in more of a male pattern of weight gain. Metabolism tends to slow down then, too. I've coined this time the *midlife metabolic crisis* because it's a normal part of life that calls for action. Lifestyle changes play a key role, though. What and how you eat make a big difference!

Revamping your eating with the Total Body Diet approach can help keep your waistline in check. Put the brakes on too much added sugar, salt, and highly processed food, and focus on the quality of your calories with whole foods like fruits, vegetables, whole grains, lowfat dairy products (like milk, cheese, and yogurt), beans, peas, nuts, seeds, and lean meats (skinless poultry and seafood).

Chapter 4

Designing a Total Body Diet–Friendly Kitchen

● ●

In This Chapter

▶ Identifying the kinds of foods you want in your kitchen

▶ Discovering simple fridge and pantry makeover tips

▶ Budgeting the Total Body Diet way

▶ Mastering meal planning and grocery shopping

● ●

A large part of living the Total Body Diet is reconfiguring your kitchen to factor in healthful foods for energy, vitality, and happiness. What foods are good for your total body? How can you figure out how to revamp your kitchen for the better and rid it of foods that are not doing your body or mind good? With simple tricks and tips for planning meals and making grocery shopping easy, you uncover ways to map out a plan that works for you and your family.

In this chapter, you get to design your kitchen to meet your Total Body Diet lifestyle. From organizing your fridge to stocking pantry essentials to smart grocery shopping tactics to planning meals and snacks, you'll feel empowered taking control of your home food environment.

Ridding Your Kitchen of Not-So-Healthy Foods

You wouldn't give your high-end, luxury car low-quality fuel, so why feed it to yourself? The Total Body Diet is about making high-quality foods a priority in your life. Before you embark on your kitchen redesign, think about the foods that don't do much good for you. Food products that are highly processed, jam-packed with added sugar, salt, and unhealthy fats — think cookies, crackers, donuts, muffins, sugary cereals, and processed meats — are not doing your body or mind any good.

Beware of some foods that are disguised as good for you, such as some brands of granola, oatmeal, or fruit bars, yogurt-covered pretzels and raisins, banana chips, trail mix, cereals, store-bought muffins, fruit cups (in syrup), light popcorn, and fruit-flavored yogurt. Read the fine print — the ingredients will reveal a lot. Also, beware of food products with partially hydrogenated vegetable oils — they most likely contain a lot of added sugar and possibly too much *trans fat* (the fats that are implicated in heart disease risk).

Your fridge

When was the last time you looked in your fridge? I mean *really* looked — moved stuff around, checked expiration dates, and realized what's good for you and what's not. It's eye-opening! I bet there are things in there that you've forgotten about or you bought in haste or used for a recipe and then buried it way in the back. The things in the front of the fridge get the most attention, so move fruits and vegetables to the front. (You don't have to use the produce cooler — especially, if you forget to look in there!)

Food kept in the fridge, should be less than 40 degrees. (Use a refrigerator thermometer to verify the temperature of your fridge.) Refrigerate perishable foods within two hours (or one hour if it's 90 degrees or hotter outside) and place foods for thawing or marinating in the bottom shelf of the refrigerator (not on the countertop). If you want extra assurance that your food is safe, check out the Home Food Safety Program's app, Is My Food Safe? and their website, www.homefoodsafety.org.

Table 4-1 has some healthy food options to stock in your fridge.

Table 4-1		**Healthy Fridge Foods**		
Whole Grains*	**Fruits**	**Vegetables**	**Proteins**	**Dairy Products/ Dairy Alternatives**
Whole-wheat flour	Applesauce (no sugar added)	Artichoke hearts	Eggs	Fat-free or lowfat milk
Whole-grain tortillas	Blueberries	Asparagus	Hummus	Kefir

Whole Grains*	Fruits	Vegetables	Proteins	Dairy Products/ Dairy Alternatives
Whole-wheat pasta	Blackberries	Beets	Tofu	Fat-free or lowfat regular or Greek yogurt (plain)
Barley	Cantaloupe	Broccoli	Nut butter (natural)	Reduced-fat or lowfat cheese
Brown rice	Cherries	Brussels sprouts	Nuts	String cheese
Bulgur wheat	Grapes	Cabbage	Bison	Reduced-fat or lowfat cottage cheese
Whole-wheat couscous	Honeydew	Carrots	Chicken breast	Farmer's cheese
Farro	Mango, sliced	Cauliflower	Chicken sausage	Butter (unsalted)
Oats	Prunes	Celery	Turkey breast	Soymilk (plain)**
Spelt	Raisins	Cucumber	Lean (95%–97%) ground sirloin	Almond milk (plain)**
Quinoa	Raspberries	Eggplant	Beef (loin and round cuts)	Hazelnut milk (plain)**
	Strawberries	Green beans	Lean roast beef	Rice milk (plain)**
	Watermelon	Hearts of palm	Ham (low fat, low sodium)	
	Fruit bowls (in their own juice)	Jicama slices	Pork loin	
		Kale		
		Kohlrabi		
		Leeks		
		Mushrooms		
		Mustard greens		

(continued)

Table 4-1 *(continued)*

Whole Grains*	Fruits	Vegetables	Proteins	Dairy Products/ Dairy Alternatives
		Okra		
		Onions		
		Pea pods		
		Peppers (all varieties)		
		Radishes		
		Romaine lettuce		
		Salsa		
		Salad greens		
		Scallions		
		Spinach		
		Summer squash		
		Tomatoes		
		Grape tomatoes		
		Turnips		
		Water chestnuts		
		Watercress		
		Zucchini		
		V-8 or tomato juice (low sodium)		

*Refined grains can have a place in your diet as they are fortified with important vitamins like the B-vitamin, folic acid, which is vital during pregnancy for the brain and spinal cord development of babies. Make half of your grains whole grains, and the rest can be refined, enriched grains.
**Shelf-stable aseptic packages require refrigeration after opening.

There are lots of veggies to choose from — aim to get 6 to 11 servings per day for overall health. Check out your fridge or grocery cart. Are you stocking enough for the week?

Don't forget to include fresh herbs and spices in your fridge. Not only are they great for boosting the healthfulness of your meals and snacks, but fresh rosemary, basil, thyme, dill, sage, and ginger, among others, offer an aromatic quality that delights the senses when you open the refrigerator door.

Keeping fresh herbs can be tricky. The hearty herbs like rosemary and thyme tend to last longer, but delicate basil, sage, and dill don't fare as well. A trick to keeping herbs fresh as long as possible is to wrap them snugly in a damp paper towel — like swaddling a baby. The leaves like the moisture — but not too much moisture, or they'll corrode quickly. Place them in the crisper drawer.

No need to refrigerate the following fruits: apple, avocado, banana, grapefruit, kiwi, clementine, orange, nectarine, papaya, peach, pear, pineapple, plum, and tangerine. You can keep them on the countertop to ripen. After you cut, bite, or peel them, it's time to refrigerate.

Your freezer

These days there's not much that can't be frozen — the only foods that you should *not* freeze are canned foods or eggs in shells. Walk down the frozen food aisles in your grocery store and you'll see a bounty of choices in every food group — from vegetables and fruits to meat, beans, and nuts to dairy products to whole grains.

There are many good reasons to stock your freezer. According to the Frozen Food Association, here are four handy facts about frozen foods:

✔ **Frozen foods are nutritious.** Frozen fruits and vegetables are flash-frozen at the highest point of nutritional value and have been found to have equal, if not more, nutrients.

Recent research from the University of California–Davis and the University of Georgia compared the nutrient content of eight commonly purchased frozen and fresh fruits and vegetables: blueberries, strawberries, corn, broccoli, cauliflower, green beans, green peas, and spinach. The University of Georgia study found that vitamins A and C and folate were greater in several frozen varieties than their fresh-stored counterparts. The University of California–Davis study found that the frozen produce preserved vitamins C and B2 better than the fresh-stored vegetables. Also, freezing the fruits and vegetables correlated to higher vitamin E levels and minerals like calcium, magnesium, zinc, copper, and iron, as well as fiber and *phytochemicals* (health-promoting compounds in plants).

✔ **Frozen foods are easy to prepare.** The best thing about frozen foods is that they come washed, precut, and ready to eat or cook. They save time and reduce waste. Plus, many are portable, convenient, simple to cook, and easy to clean up, all of which bodes well for time-pressed families.

✔ **Frozen foods are a real value.** Not only do frozen foods stretch your food dollars, but they deliver on quality and taste, offering real consumer value. Plus, frozen foods have a much greater shelf life than refrigerated foods, allowing easier portioning and storing to use at a later date.

✔ **Frozen foods are the sensible choice.** From a calorie-control standpoint, frozen foods offer many pre-portioned options, as well as resealable packaging to take out a portion and save the rest. Plus, they take the guesswork out by providing nutrition facts on the label.

Table 4-2 offers healthy food options to stock in your freezer (at 0 degrees or below).

Table 4-2		Healthy Freezer Foods		
Whole Grains	**Fruits**	**Vegetables**	**Proteins**	**Dairy Products/Dairy Alternatives**
Whole-wheat flour	Bananas	Artichoke hearts	Nuts	Kefir
Whole-wheat breads	Blackberries	Asparagus	Bison	Fat-free or lowfat regular or Greek yogurt
Whole-grain tortillas	Blueberries	Beets	Chicken breast	Ice milk
Brown rice, precooked	Cantaloupe	Broccoli	Chicken sausage	Lowfat ice cream
Wild rice, precooked	Cherries	Brussels sprouts	Turkey breast	
	Grapes	Cabbage	Lean (95%–97%) ground sirloin	
	Honeydew	Carrots	Beef (loin and round cuts)	
	Mango, sliced	Cauliflower	Lean roast beef	

Whole Grains	Fruits	Vegetables	Proteins	Dairy Products/Dairy Alternatives
	Raspberries	Celery	Ham (lowfat, low sodium)	
	Strawberries	Chili	Pork loin	
	Watermelon	Cucumber		
	Pureed fruit pops	Eggplant		
	Fruit sorbet	Green beans		
		Hearts of palm		
		Jicama slices		
		Kale		
		Kohlrabi		
		Leeks		
		Mustard greens		
		Okra		
		Onions		
		Pea pods		
		Peppers (all varieties)		
		Radishes		
		Salsa		
		Scallions		
		Summer squash		
		Sweet potatoes (fries)		
		Tomato sauce		
		Turnips		
		Water chestnuts		
		Zucchini		

Frozen, prepared meals are convenient and portion controlled, but be sure to check the Nutrition Facts label and ingredients for sodium, added sources of sugar, saturated fat, and trans fat.

Label and date foods before putting them in the freezer. You can download and print out handy freezer labels at `www.homefoodsafety.org/downloads/food-safety-freezer-labels`.

Your pantry

The pantry cupboards are often forgotten because they house the shelf-stable, nonperishable foods that can last through the next Ice Age — or so you think. Cleaning out your pantry doesn't have to just happen in springtime. Any time of year works for tossing outdated dried herbs and spices, old boxes of clumped-together raisins, aging vegetable oils, and stale crackers. Organizing the shelves, dusting off cans, and taking stock of what's in the dark recesses of your pantry is liberating.

Here are some tips for your pantry makeover:

- ✔ Keep it clean, cool (50 to 70 degrees), dry, and dark.
- ✔ Check the dates on boxes, cans, and bags of dried goods.
- ✔ Place older products up front to use first.
- ✔ Discard any bulging, cracked, or dented cans (because there's a risk of botulism lurking in the damaged can).
- ✔ Discard dried herbs and spices after one year (because their beneficial compounds and flavors diminish after this point). Be sure to put a purchase date on the container.
- ✔ Store open pasta, rice, and flour in an air-tight container to keep away rodents or insects.

Table 4-3 lists healthy food options to stock in your pantry.

Table 4-3	Healthy Pantry Foods		
Whole Grains	*Fruits*	*Vegetables*	*Proteins*
Unopened whole-wheat flour (in an airtight container)	Canned fruits (no sugar added)	Canned vegetables (no salt added)	Nuts (in an airtight container)

Whole Grains	Fruits	Vegetables	Proteins
Whole-wheat breads	Dried fruits (could also refrigerate)	Beans	Tuna fish*
Brown rice		Lentils	Salmon*
Wild rice		Soups	Crabmeat*
Whole-grain pasta		Potatoes (with skin)	Sardines
Couscous		Sweet potatoes (with skin)	Shrimp*
Quinoa		Peas	Chicken*
Popcorn		Corn	Soymilk (plain)**
High-fiber cereals		Vegetarian chili	Almond milk**
Oatmeal		Bean dip	Hazelnut milk**
			Rice milk**

*Cans/pouches (in water)
**In aseptic cartons

Cooking Techniques for Your Total Body

The way you cook food is just as important as the food itself. Take a potato, for instance. In its plain form, it's a nutritious food — high in vitamin C and potassium with no sodium or fat. Bake it and pierce it open and fill it with broccoli and a drizzle of olive oil and dash of salt and pepper, and the health benefits shine. On the other hand, slice it and deep-fry it in a vat of oil and douse it with salt, and the healthy side is masked by a high-calorie glaze of fat.

One goal of the Total Body Diet is to make the healthy side of foods shine bright in your life! Using cooking techniques that enable this to happen is important, so in this section I give you a close-up look at these culinary methods in action.

Grilling

According to the Hearth, Patio, and Barbecue Association (HPBA), practically everyone grills. Eighty percent of U.S. households own a grill or smoker — and 97 percent of them used the grill within the last year!

The taste of grilled foods is the number one reason that grilling is so hot these days. It's a healthier way to cook because grilling drains the fat from meats and they aren't battered or sitting in grease. Plus, grilling offers the opportunity to make vegetables — think kabobs, as well as steamer baskets filled with colorful arrays of veggies.

Charring the flesh of meat, fish, chicken, or pork can produce potentially *carcinogenic* (cancer-causing) compounds called heterocyclic amines and polycyclic aromatic hydrocarbons. The good news is, marinating the flesh of any of these meats will hinder the production of these compounds. To play it safe, don't overcook grilled meats, and flip meat on the grill often.

Here are some healthier grilling tactics:

- **Grill veggies and fruits.** Adding some colorful foods to the barbecue will provide fiber and antioxidants. Plus, grilled produce doesn't form the cancer-causing compounds that charred meats do. Some great produce to grill are mushrooms, potatoes, tomatoes, onions, zucchini, yellow squash, eggplant, apples, pears, and pineapples.

- **Alternate meat with plants.** Grilling high-fat meats is not a good practice for heart health and your waistline. Instead, use leaner loin cuts of beef and pork and skinless chicken breast — and don't forget the plants! It's easy to skewer tofu on a kabob with zucchini, onions, and tomatoes. Portobello mushrooms make a great grilled food on a whole-grain bun (and they taste like meat!). Veggie burgers are tasty on the grill, too.

- **Whip up some healthy marinades.** Not only do marinades offer protection from chemical compounds forming on meat, but if you make them with less fat, it reduces the fat drippings in the fire forming the compounds in the first place. Use vinegar, lemon or lime juice, honey, garlic, herbs, and spices.

Roasting

You can roast everything from vegetables to fruits to meats to nuts to beans to spices like coriander and cumin seeds. The best part about roasting is that it imparts such great flavor. Roasting uses dry heat to cook and brown the exterior of the foods, forming complex flavors and scents. The beauty of roasting is that you can set the food in the oven and do other things while it's cooking.

Less is more when it comes to roasting. Nuts taste lovely roasted raw. Elephant garlic requires a drizzle of olive oil and a dash of salt. Root vegetables roast well with a bit of olive oil, smoked paprika, salt, and pepper.

Broiling

Unlike grilling, food is heated from above with broiling. This cooking method saves time because the high heat from the broiler expedites the cooking process. Plus, broiling can happen in any weather and it offers faster prep and cleanup.

Here are some fun and tasty ways to use your broiler:

- ✔ Seared tofu with mushrooms and green onions
- ✔ Melted cheese sandwich with tomatoes
- ✔ Chicken quesadilla with cheddar and chipotle peppers

Sautéing

Browning food in a hot pan with a little fat is the gist of a good sauté. It's a common culinary technique worldwide. From mushrooms, onions, and garlic (my favorite combo) to chicken, beef, or pork, sautéing is a convenient way to cook because it requires only a stovetop and a small skillet (or sauté pan).

Here are a few key things to think about for healthier sautéing:

- ✔ **Choose a healthier fat.** Good options include canola or grapeseed oil (because they have a higher smoke point and can withstand high heat).
- ✔ **Stir often.** Foods can burn in the sauté pan, if you aren't careful — especially minced garlic and other herbs.
- ✔ **Don't overdo the oil — a little goes a long way.** A tablespoon of oil is 120 calories, so use it sparingly. A good tip is to pour a bit in and spread with a paper towel — that way, excess oil will be absorbed.

Steaming

Using steam heat to cook is low in both fat and calories. Plus, it's a short cooking method — a few minutes is all you need. Unlike boiling, where you submerse a food in water, with steaming you don't lose as much of the nutrients. If anything, there's evidence that steaming can help bring out the nutritional value in vegetables.

Research in the *Journal of the Science of Food and Agriculture* found that steaming was the best method for preserving phytochemicals in plant-based foods.

Every vegetable requires a unique steaming time depending on its weight and cell structure. Delicate leafy greens will be heated through quickly, whereas hearty broccoli, cauliflower, and Brussels sprouts will take longer. Keep that in mind and group vegetables together based on their unique cooking needs.

Baking

One of the first cooking methods on Earth, baking uses prolonged heat from the oven. Food is cooked from the outside to the center. You typically think of bread, cookies, and cakes with baking, but you can bake meat, poultry, fish, pizza, casseroles, potatoes, and vegetables.

Similar to roasting, baking doesn't require a lot of work. You just pop it in the oven and do other things while your meal is cooking. Plus, it's a lowfat cooking method as you don't need to use fat to bake. (Of course, baked sweet goods contain fat, so limit cookies and cakes!)

Microwaving

It doesn't seem like it would be healthy to put food in a box and bombard it with electromagnetic radiation to cook it, but there's nothing to say it's not.

To the contrary, research has shown that foods retain their nutrient content after microwaving just the same as with other cooking methods, if not better. Quick cooking time may actually preserve nutritional value, and some research has shown that folate levels in leafy greens like spinach are better preserved when microwaved versus cooked on the stovetop.

Here are the benefits of microwaving:

- It's quick and easy and the cleanup is minimal.
- It preserves nutrients better than other cooking methods that take longer and use more liquid.
- Many healthy foods are microwaveable, such as vegetables, chicken, fish, pasta, rice, quinoa, and couscous dishes. Microwaving is a convenient way to get a varied, nutrient-rich diet.

Eating Well on a Budget

It doesn't have to cost a lot to eat well. You'll be surprised how much money you save if you eliminate mindless eating. By planning meals and snacks and purchasing food at regular times, your grocery bills will become more streamlined.

Earlier in this chapter, I talk about frozen foods — they're one of the best ways to stretch your food dollars. Frozen produce, meats, fish, beans, and even grains go a longer way. However, there are healthy and cheap ways to eat, dine out, cook for more than one occasion, as well as shop the grocery store with your budget in mind.

Healthy and cheap eats

Food doesn't have to be gourmet or break your budget to be healthy. Simple, whole foods top the health charts — and you can bargain-shop for it. An example of healthy and cheap is eating meatless. You don't have to be a vegan or vegetarian to follow the Total Body Diet, but at least one day a week, try going without meat and eat plant-based meals instead. Your heart, blood sugar, blood pressure, and waistline will thank you later!

Here are some simple cheap eats to put on your list:

- ✔ **Tofu (soybean curd):** Extra-firm is good to make stir-fries and baked with a marinade.
- ✔ **Tempeh (fermented soybeans):** Add to salads or chili or enjoy it solo with vegetables.
- ✔ **Beans:** Black, kidney, navy, pinto, lima, or garbanzo.
- ✔ **Lentils:** Red, green, or brown.
- ✔ **Quinoa (pronounced keen-wah):** A high-protein grain to add to salads, soups, chili, and stir-fries.

Cook once, eat twice

Leftovers are one of greatest time-saving and budgeting techniques. When you prepare a meal, make more than you need for just one meal. For example, bake more chicken breasts than you need and refrigerate the rest for the next day to shred into tacos or chili. Double your soup recipe or cut up more vegetables than you need to have on hand for the next day's meals.

Make a meal plan for the week and identify where you could cook once and enjoy it for a couple of meals. For example, you might end up with something like this:

Monday	Tuesday	Wednesday	Thursday	Friday	Saturday	Sunday
Bake chicken	Chicken tacos	Grilled portobello mushroom and veggie wrap	Mushroom and greens salad	Stir-fry tofu	Toss tofu into soup	Tofu scramble
Chili						

Savvy grocery store shopping

Let's face it: You're in the grocery store frequently, or else you avoid it like the plague. Either way, there's a better path. By becoming more focused on planning, your grocery shopping experiences will improve. According to the USDA (www.choosemyplate.gov/budget), there are a number of places where you can go to save money while buying good-quality food:

- ✔ Regular grocery stores
- ✔ Ethnic markets
- ✔ Dollar stores
- ✔ Retail supercenters
- ✔ Wholesale clubs
- ✔ Farmer's markets

Although it may not seem realistic to store-hop, you may find better prices on eggs and milk at one store, but better prices on produce at another. If you plan your trips with a list, you can schedule to shop at different stores on set days.

Here are some grocery shopping organization tips:

- ✔ Keep a running grocery list and jot down what you run out of as you go through the week.
- ✔ Clip coupons and take advantage of the store's flyer deals.
- ✔ Buy store brands — they offer good-quality food at a cheaper price.

Planning Your Meals for Success

Planning is one of the anchoring principles of eating well on a budget, according to the USDA. (The other two are purchasing and preparing.) How does your eating success hinge on establishing a weekly eating game plan? It's not rocket science, but following a food plan not only helps you with your financial budget, but also helps you save calories.

Becoming a meal-planning pro

Think of yourself as a meal planner in training. You may not think it now, but in no time you'll become a meal-planning pro, if you start small and build from there. Here are some key things you can do in order to stay on top of your meals for the week ahead:

- Use online recipes, message boards, and apps for inspiration.
- Participate in a recipe exchange with friends, neighbors, or co-workers.
- Add ingredients for new recipes to your grocery list.
- Keep your meals simple with four or five ingredients maximum. There are many great cookbooks using minimal ingredients. Check out *Best Ever Three & Four Ingredient Cookbook,* by Jenny White and Joanna Farrow, or *The Four Ingredient Cookbook,* by Linda Coffee and Emily Cale.

Set it and forget it

Now that you have a plan, you can prepare ahead of time or even do a quick prep that day. When you've mapped it out in your head, there's no guesswork and you can save time. If you have to leave for the day, you can put a meal in a slow cooker and let it cook all day. Then it'll be ready when you get home!

The forget-it part of this equation allows you to get other things done without running around last minute to throw a meal together or just stopping at a fast-food place on the way home because you don't have any idea what to eat for dinner.

You can make everything from oatmeal to curries to chili to pork to beef to chicken dishes to pasta sauces in a slow cooker. There are literally hundreds of recipes. For inspiration, check out *Slow Cookers For Dummies,* by Tom Lacalamita and Glenna Vance (Wiley).

Navigating grocery store trips

You can streamline grocery store trips simply by having a list and visualizing the store. Categorize the foods that you need — such as fruits and vegetables, chicken, fish, eggs, milk, breads, and cereals — and map out the best path to fill your cart.

Before you shop, eat something — you'll be more prone to make impulse purchases if you're hungry.

Shop the perimeter of the grocery store first — that's where you'll most likely find fresh produce, whole-grain breads, meat, and dairy items.

Compare and save by looking at the unit price of items — not the actual price. The unit price is the total price per unit. The lower the price per unit, the better the deal. Many grocery stores list the price per unit on the shelf price tag, so you can compare prices more easily.

Purchase frozen items to save money, but be sure to check for added sugar, salt, and fat. Buying family packs saves money, but be sure to refrigerate or freeze remaining portions, such as meats, cheeses, pastas, rice, and breads.

Skip the chip and cookie aisle to save money (and excess calories from entering your home!). Also, plan to make homemade cookies as a treat. This way you can throw healthier ingredients in, too.

Avoid buying sugar-laden beverages. Instead, purchase a reusable water bottle and use filtered tap water. You'll save money and calories in the long run.

For more grocery shopping tips, recipes, and food budgeting ideas, check out What's Cooking? The USDA's Mixing Bowl at www.whatscooking.fns. usda.gov.

Part II
Total Body Diet Rules

Five Fantastic Ways to Listen to Your Total Body

- **Use your noggin.** When you think about your overall health, keeping your brain fueled well should be first and foremost in your mind. Your brain is the largest organ in your body and is fueled well with good-quality carbohydrates like whole fruit, vegetables, and grains, plus beneficial fats like omega-3 fatty acids found in fish and walnuts and flax, chia, and hemp seeds.

- **Flex your muscles.** If you often feel sluggish or tired, ask yourself whether you're getting enough exercise. Aim to get physical activity regularly by walking, biking, running, or swimming at least 150 minutes a week. Stretching is also a great way to keep muscles flexible and happy.

- **Re-energize with nutrient-dense foods.** Foods that give you extended amounts of energy throughout the day are also great for your overall health. For meals, fill up half of your plate with colorful produce from vegetables and fruits; a quarter of your plate with powerful proteins from lean red meat, skinless poultry, fish, tofu, beans, or legumes; and the other quarter with grains (half of the time whole grains like whole wheat, quinoa, brown rice, and/or oats).

- **Hydrate with water.** Drink plenty of fluids — and preferably beverages without a lot of calories, such as water, unsweetened tea, and black coffee. The amount of fluid you need depends on your gender, age, and activity level. The more you sweat, the more water you'll need to replenish fluid losses.

- **Give yourself a break.** If you have a day of not eating well or you forget to drink water, aim to get back on the healthy habits horse at the earliest opportunity. You can choose more wisely at the next meal or drink a glass of water before you leave the office or go out for the evening. Don't be hard on yourself — just keep forging ahead.

Find out why fad diets don't work in a free article at www.dummies.com/extras/totalbodydiet.

In this part . . .

- ✔ Get a brief overview of the total body diet approach.
- ✔ Learn what foods to focus on for total body wellness.
- ✔ Understand what calories are and how to portion-control them.
- ✔ Set the bar higher for your physical activity goals to keep weight gain at bay.
- ✔ Put a team in place to support your total body wellness goals.

Chapter 5

Foods for Total Body Balance

. . . .

In This Chapter

▶ Homing in on beneficial food choices for your Total Body Diet plan

▶ Understanding the three big nutrients: carbohydrates, proteins, and fats

▶ Maximizing nutritional value on your plate while allowing small indulgences

. . . .

*H*ealthy foods can be medicinal — they can keep your body and mind in tip-top shape and actually increase the quality *and* quantity of your life. To the contrary, eating too many highly processed foods with a lot of added sugar, sodium, and solid fat can increase the risk of chronic diseases like obesity, type-2 diabetes, heart disease, and certain cancers.

The Centers for Disease Control and Prevention (CDC) reports that more than one-third of adults in the United States are obese. In a world where fast, convenient food is everywhere, this is not surprising. The good news is, you can make changes today in your eating and lifestyle that can make a significant health difference and lead to weight loss, as well as reduce the risk of diseases (or delay their progression) down the road.

It's all about balancing your days to the best of your eating ability by adding healthy foods in, whenever you can. Most of the day, choose fruits and vegetables, lean proteins, whole grains, and fat-free and lowfat dairy. When you eat your favorite comfort foods, add a nutritional boost:

✔ Top pizza and pasta with vegetables or have a side salad with it.

✔ Mix onions, mushrooms, garlic, oregano, and dry oats into ground beef for a nutrient-packed burger or meatloaf.

✔ Savor a piece of dark chocolate instead of milk chocolate (which has more sugar and saturated fat).

✔ Add sliced fruit like strawberries, peaches, or apples, and a dash of cinnamon to a scoop of lowfat plain yogurt.

In this chapter, I explain which foods are beneficial for total body wellness. I cover everything from what to stock in your pantry and fridge to how to inspect food labels for ingredients like added sugars, fats, and sodium.

Identifying the Primary Players: Carbs, Protein, and Fat

This question has been lurking for decades: What is the right balance of nutrients? Your body and mind function best when you give them a balance of the three macronutrients: carbohydrate, protein, and fat. Because each of us has unique nutritional needs, the Institute of Medicine (IOM) recommends a daily healthy range for each of the macronutrients for adults:

- **Carbohydrates:** 45 percent to 65 percent

- **Protein:** 10 percent to 35 percent

- **Fat:** 20 percent to 35 percent

Think about it, are you getting too many carbs and not enough protein or too much protein and not enough fat? Let's delve more deeply into each of the macronutrients and see how to balance them every day in a healthful way.

Carbohydrates

Carbohydrates hold a special place in the diet as they are the main energy source for the brain and they provide glucose (blood sugar) to every cell in the body. Although carbohydrates come from a variety of foods that are good for you, as well as foods that are not so good for you, the whole group takes the heat by many commercial weight loss diet plans. Let's set your path to total body wellness straight; you need carbs to live, breathe, think, work, and play. Carbs are important for living a quality life, but choosing the better-for-you carbs in the right quantities — *most* of the time — is the key.

Here's a list of nutrient-dense carbs (which you should choose from daily):

- **Fruits:** Apples, bananas, berries, clementines, grapes, oranges, mangoes, and so on

- **Vegetables:** Artichokes, asparagus, broccoli, Brussels sprouts, cauliflower, green beans, mushrooms, spinach, and so on

✔ **Beans and peas:** Black beans, chickpeas or garbanzo beans, pinto beans, navy beans, Lima beans, cannellini beans, lentils, and so on

✔ **Whole grains:** Whole wheat bread and crackers, whole wheat pasta, brown rice, quinoa, millet, farro, oatmeal, plain popcorn, and so on

✔ **Fat-free and lowfat dairy:** Skim and lowfat milk; Swiss, provolone, and part-skim mozzarella; plain lowfat yogurt

Less-healthy carbs, which you can eat occasionally, include the following:

✔ Baked goods with added sugar and solid fat (for example, cakes, cookies, some breads, muffins, doughnuts, croissants)

✔ Candy, lollipops, gummy candies

✔ Beverages with added sugar, like soft drinks, sweetened juice beverages, and sweetened tea and coffee drinks

✔ Chips (for example, potato chips, corn chips, tortilla chips)

✔ Crackers (for example, white flour crackers)

✔ Cheese and caramel popcorn

In the following sections, I walk you through the good kinds of carbohydrates in greater detail.

Whole-grain goodness

A *whole grain* contains 100 percent of the original kernel — all of the bran, germ, and endosperm — even if the grain has been processed, such as cracked, crushed, rolled, extruded, and/or cooked. Why are whole grains so good for you? Whole grains are jam-packed with dietary fiber, which may help reduce blood cholesterol levels and the risk of heart disease, type-2 diabetes, and obesity, as well as fend off constipation. Keep in mind, fiber-rich foods like whole grains can fill you up on fewer calories and may help with weight management. Whole grains contain numerous other vitamins and minerals, such as iron, B vitamins (folate, niacin, thiamin, and riboflavin), magnesium, and selenium.

The Dietary Guidelines for Americans (2010) recommends that at least half of your grains contain the whole grain as opposed to refined grains like white flour, de-germed cornmeal, white bread, and white rice. Are you getting at least three servings of whole grains every day? Studies show that over 40 percent of Americans never eat whole grains at all, according to the Whole Grains Council.

The following are all examples of a serving of whole grain:

- ✔ One slice of whole-grain bread
- ✔ 1 cup ready-to-eat whole grain cereal
- ✔ ½ cup cooked brown rice, whole-wheat pasta, or oatmeal
- ✔ One mini whole-grain bagel
- ✔ ½ cup cooked bulgur
- ✔ ½ whole-wheat English muffin
- ✔ 3 cups popped popcorn
- ✔ 1 small (6-inch) whole-grain tortilla
- ✔ 2 small (3-inch) whole-wheat pancakes

The amount of grains you need daily depends on your age, sex, and level of physical activity. In other words, the more active you are, the more grains you may be able to eat and stay within your calorie allotment for the day.

Check labels for whole grains. If it says "whole wheat" on the front of the package, read the ingredient list. Look for the word *whole* before *wheat* or *grain* as the first ingredient listed to ensure that it's a whole-grain product. If it says "enriched wheat," it's a refined-grain product (but B vitamins and iron are added back in, which is good). Fiber is not added back in, however, so it's not a fiber-rich food. Many grain products are a mixture of whole and refined grains.

You can also check the label for a whole grains stamp (created by the Whole Grains Council) to signify that it's a whole-grain product. There are two stamps: products marked with the 100% Whole Grain stamp contain a full serving of whole grains or 16 grams of whole grain per serving; those marked with the Whole Grain stamp contain a half serving of whole grains or 8 grams of whole grains per serving. Remember, for many people, the recommended amount of whole grains per day is a minimum of three servings or 48 grams of whole grains.

Not every whole-grain product contains the Whole Grains stamp. It's a voluntary stamp for manufacturers to use at their discretion and own cost. So examining food labels carefully is the real sure-fire way to detect if a food is made from whole grains.

Pulses: Beans, lentils, and peas

Pulses are a type of legume or seeds that grow within pods. Beans and peas are the mature form of legumes. Examples are garbanzo beans, black beans, kidney beans, pinto beans, black-eyed peas, split peas, and lentils.

Green peas and green lima beans are different and are grouped with starchy vegetables (such as corn and potatoes). Green (string) beans are considered non-starchy vegetables like onions, lettuce, celery, and cabbage.

Pulses offer distinct health benefits. The USDA Food Patterns classify them as both vegetables *and* protein food sources. Like other vegetables, pulses are an excellent source of fiber and contain plant-based nutrients like the B vitamin folate, as well as potassium, which helps regulate blood pressure. The Dietary Guidelines for Americans recommends frequent consumption of peas and beans because they offer plant-based health benefits, such as helping to reduce the risk of heart disease, type-2 diabetes, obesity, and certain cancers. Plus, they're also great meat, poultry, and fish alternatives because they contain plant-based sources of protein, iron, and zinc. For vegetarians and vegans, a variety of plants are recommended because most beans and peas are not complete protein sources.

Look at your eating patterns to factor in where beans and peas can fit into your diet for total body balance. If you eat meat, poultry, and fish, you can count beans and peas as vegetables. In general, adults should eat 1½ to 2 cups of beans and peas per week. Look here to see your needs: www.choosemyplate.gov/food-groups/vegetables-amount.pdf.

If you're vegan or vegetarian or you eat animal protein very seldom, you can count beans and peas as some of your protein source. In general, adults should eat 5 to 6½ ounces of protein per day. Look here to see your needs: www.choosemyplate.gov/food-groups/protein-foods-amount.pdf.

One serving of beans and peas consists of any of the following:

- ¼ cup of cooked beans, peas, refried beans, and baked beans counts as a 1-ounce equivalent of protein.
- 1 cup of cooked, whole or mashed beans and peas counts as 1 cup of vegetables.

Fantastic fruits

Who doesn't love the sweetness of a ripe, juicy piece of fruit? Not only is fruit packed with water, but it's jam-packed with antioxidants for cell health — from vitamin C in oranges, grapefruit, kiwi, limes, and lemons, to carotenoids like lycopene in tomatoes and watermelon, which may help aid in cancer defense (primarily prostate cancer in men), to fiber like pectin in apples, apricots, pears, plums, and citrus fruits, which helps alleviate diarrhea and constipation.

Your total body wellness relies on a daily dose of fruit. With the MyPlate recommendation to make half of your plate fruits and vegetables, it's important to factor fruit in at meals and snacks. The goal for adults is 1½ to 2 cups of fruit every day. Fruit comes in all shapes and sizes, so Table 5-1 explains what constitutes one serving of some common fruits. For more, check out www.choosemyplate.gov/food-groups/fruits-foodgallery.html.

Table 5-1	Serving Sizes of Various Fruits
Type of Fruit	*One Serving Equals . . .*
Apple	One small apple (2½ inches in diameter) or 1 cup sliced
Banana	One large banana (8 to 9 inches long) or 1 cup sliced
Cantaloupe	1 cup diced or melon balls
Grapes	1 cup whole or cut up, approximately 32 seedless grapes
Grapefruit	1 cup sections or one medium (4-inch diameter) grapefruit
Peach	1 large (2¾-inch diameter) peach
Strawberries	8 large berries or 1 cup whole, halved, or sliced
Dried fruit	½ cup raisins, prunes, or apricots
100% fruit juice*	1 cup

If you can, eat the whole fruit instead of drinking the juice — you'll fill up on more fiber and chewing allows you to eat it more slowly and mindfully.

Fruit offers a whole host of culinary opportunities, whether fresh, frozen, canned (in its 100 percent fruit juice or water), cooked, or pureed. Here are some delicious ways to get fruit on your plate every day:

- ✔ Toss frozen berries into plain lowfat yogurt with ground flaxseed and a dash of cinnamon, and puree into a smoothie.

- ✔ Top a slice of whole-grain toast with sliced apples and peanut butter.

- ✔ Chop fresh mangos, tomatoes, onions, and cilantro to make a salsa.

- ✔ Cook fresh cranberries, cinnamon, and nutmeg with honey or agave nectar (a natural sweetener from the agave plant) to make a delicious cranberry sauce.

- ✔ Sprinkle raisins over a mixed green salad with sliced strawberries and avocado.

- ✔ Top cooked oatmeal with blueberries or raspberries with some chopped walnuts or pistachios.

If you can't find organic fruit or it's too pricey for your budget, buy the conventionally grown varieties and wash and scrub it — even the skins and rinds that you don't eat — with a produce brush under cold, running tap water.

Valuable veggies

From dark, leafy greens to red, orange, and yellow hues, the vegetable family's wide array of colors do your total body good. The plant compounds inherent in the flesh, skins, and stalks and stems, as well as the fiber, vitamins, and minerals in vegetables have shown to help reduce the risk of heart disease and various forms of cancer. A recent review of several studies in the *British Journal of Nutrition* found that beyond reduced risk of heart disease, regularly eating vegetables (and fruits) reduced the risk of several cancers — specifically in the digestive tract. So that's all the more reason to get your veggies!

Eating vegetables can keep your waistline in check, too. They're low-calorie and packed with nutrients and fiber that help you fill up on fewer calories. For example, a cup of raw, chopped broccoli contains a mere 30 calories, no saturated fat, little sodium, lots of vitamin C, as well as numerous plant compounds that may help to fend off certain cancers and heart disease and boost immunity.

Whether you eat them raw, frozen, canned, dried, or dehydrated, vegetables should top your Total Body Diet plan. Adults should aim for a minimum of 2 to 3 cups of vegetables a day. The Dietary Guidelines for Americans classifies the different veggies into five subgroups: dark green, red and orange, beans and peas, starchy, and other vegetables.

A serving of vegetables is equal to 1 cup of raw or cooked vegetables or vegetable juice or 2 cups of raw leafy greens. Table 5-2 spells it out in greater detail.

Get creative with vegetables in the kitchen in the following ways:

- Toss diced tomatoes, peppers, onions, and beans into a chili.
- Chop cucumbers, tomatoes, onions, and drizzle with 1 tablespoon extra-virgin olive oil and balsamic vinegar for a tasty salad.
- Dice mushrooms, onions, and garlic and fold into eggs for an omelet.
- Puree pumpkin, onions, cinnamon, and nutmeg into a hearty soup.
- Bake a half acorn squash and drizzle with 1 tablespoon olive oil, honey, and cinnamon.

Table 5-2	Serving Sizes of Various Vegetables
Type of Vegetable	**One Serving Equals . . .**
Dark green vegetables	
Broccoli	1 cup
Greens (collards, mustard greens, turnip greens, kale)	1 cup
Raw leafy greens (spinach, romaine, watercress, dark green leafy lettuce, endive, escarole)	1 cup, cooked or 2 cups, raw
Red and orange vegetables	
Carrots	1 cup, chopped, sliced raw, or cooked, or 12 baby carrots
Pumpkin	1 cup mashed, cooked
Red pepper	1 cup chopped, raw, or cooked
Tomatoes	1 cup chopped or sliced, raw, canned, or cooked
Tomato juice	1 cup
Sweet potato	1 large baked or 1 cup, sliced or mashed, cooked
Winter squash	1 cup, cubed, cooked
Beans and peas	1/4 cup, cooked
Starchy vegetables	
Corn	1 cup or 1 large ear (8 to 9 inches long)
Green peas	1 cup, diced or mashed
White potatoes	1 medium (2½ to 3 inches diameter), boiled or baked
Other vegetables	
Bean sprouts	1 cup, cooked
Cabbage, green	1 cup shredded, raw or cooked
Cauliflower	1 cup pieces or florets, cooked or raw
Celery	1 cup diced or sliced, cooked or raw, or 2 large stalks (11 to 12 inches)

Type of Vegetable	One Serving Equals . . .
Cucumbers	1 cup raw, sliced or chopped
Green or wax beans	1 cup cooked
Green peppers	1 cup chopped, raw or cooked
Lettuce, iceberg or head	2 cups raw, shredded or chopped
Mushrooms	1 cup, raw or cooked
Onions	1 cup chopped, raw or cooked
Summer squash or zucchini	1 cup cooked, sliced or diced

A dose of dairy

Dairy products are the main source of calcium in the American diet, according to the Dietary Guidelines for Americans. The key is choosing lowfat or fat-free options to decrease calories and saturated fat. Milk, cheese, and yogurt are all dairy foods that can benefit your total body wellness. Dairy foods contain protein, calcium, vitamin D, and potassium, which are beneficial nutrients.

Non-dairy soymilk fits into the dairy group because it's calcium-fortified. Look for plain, unsweetened varieties of soymilk to decrease added sugars and empty calories.

For optimal health, get at least 3 cups a day of dairy foods. They've been linked to reduced risk of heart disease, type-2 diabetes, and lower blood pressure. In addition, the calcium and vitamin D–fortified dairy foods like milk, some yogurts, and soymilk are great for building and maintaining bone mass; plus, the potassium in these foods is fantastic for helping to keep your blood pressure in a healthy range.

Although cream cheese, sour cream, and butter are made from milk, they aren't grouped with dairy foods as they contain very little to no calcium or other dairy-related nutritional benefits. Plus, they can contain a lot of saturated fat, which can pose a risk for heart disease.

How do you get your 3 cups of dairy a day? Aim for lowfat, reduced-fat, or fat-free varieties of the foods in Table 5-3.

Table 5-3	Serving Sizes of Various Dairy Foods
Dairy Food	**One Serving Equals . . .**
Lowfat or fat-free milk	1 cup
Lowfat or fat-free yogurt	1 cup (8 ounces)
Hard cheese (cheddar, Parmesan, Swiss, and mozzarella)	1½ ounces
Shredded cheese	⅓ cup
Ricotta cheese	½ cup
Cottage cheese	2 cups
Ice cream	1½ cups
Frozen yogurt	1 cup
Pudding made with milk	1 cup
Soymilk (calcium fortified)	1 cup

If you don't eat dairy , take advantage of the many nondairy food options that can provide you with calcium:

- ✔ Calcium-fortified juices
- ✔ Calcium-fortified cereals and breads
- ✔ Canned fish like sardines and salmon with bones
- ✔ Soy products, such as tofu (made with calcium sulfate), tempeh, and soy yogurt
- ✔ Leafy greens like collards, turnip greens, kale, and bok choy

Adults should get 1,000 to 1,200 mg of calcium per day. It's simple to decipher how much calcium you're getting — just look at the food label. For example, if a cup of yogurt contains 30 percent calcium, just replace the percent sign with a zero, and you know it has 300 mg of calcium per cup.

Here are some ways to get dairy into your day:

- ✔ Cook up some oatmeal with fat-free milk and top with sliced fruit or berries.
- ✔ Enjoy a cup of plain, lowfat yogurt with berries and nuts on top.
- ✔ Pair a piece of whole-grain toast and nut butter with a glass of lowfat milk.

✔ Melt part-skim mozzarella cheese over broccoli spears for a tasty snack.

✔ Puree soymilk with assorted fruits and vegetables for a delicious smoothie.

Proteins

Protein has become the go-to nutrient these days. Although it's important to eat enough protein, some adults need to increase their protein intake while others are already getting plenty. Meat, poultry, and eggs are the most commonly consumed protein sources, while seafood, beans, peas, soy products, nuts, and seeds are eaten in smaller amounts, according to the Dietary Guidelines for Americans. For total body wellness, eating a variety of lean protein sources is your best bet.

From plants to animals, protein fuels muscle as well as offers vital nutrients and health benefits. For example, eating nuts has been associated with a lower risk of death from all causes — cancer, cardiovascular disease, respiratory disease, diabetes, neurodegenerative diseases (like dementia and Alzheimer's disease), and other causes — in a large study published in the *International Journal of Epidemiology,* which looked at 120,852 men and women ages 55 to 69 years in the Netherlands over a ten-year period. In this study, the subjects who ate tree nuts (for example, pistachios, walnuts, and almonds) and peanuts on a daily basis showed a lower risk of death from these diseases.

How much protein should you eat every day? Like all foods, it depends on your age, sex, and activity levels, but in general adults need 5½ ounces to 6 ounces of protein foods per day. How can you reach your daily recommendations without missing out or not having enough?

In the following sections, I fill you in on the different types of protein and how the servings add up to a day's worth of protein power.

Plant protein power

Plant foods are amazing — they can offer protein to power your total body for the better! Not only do plant proteins like beans, peas, nuts, seeds, soy foods (like tofu, tempeh, and edamame), and many vegetarian products offer oodles of protein, but they're also low in saturated fat and cholesterol and high in fiber, as well as plant-based compounds that may help fend of inflammation and chronic diseases (like cancer, diabetes, and heart disease), and fill you up on fewer calories.

What does a serving of plant protein look like? Table 5-4 has the answers.

Table 5-4	Serving Sizes of Various Plant Proteins
Plant Protein	*One Serving Equals . . .*
Nuts and seeds	½ ounce
Nut butter	1 tablespoon
Beans, peas, soybeans	¼ cup
Tofu	¼ cup
Tempeh	1 ounce, cooked
Falafel patty	4 ounces
Hummus	2 tablespoons

If you're a vegetarian, instead of adding high-fat cheeses for additional protein, use lowfat varieties of cheese, Greek yogurt (because it's higher in protein than regular yogurt), milk, soymilk, and tofu.

Protein from land and sea

From red meat to poultry to pork to seafood, protein is highest in animal foods. Animal protein offers all the essential *amino acids* (building blocks of muscles and cells). On the downside, you need to choose your animal protein wisely because certain cuts of beef, pork, and the dark meat of chicken and turkey are high in saturated fat. Trim all visible fat and marbling in red meat or pork, and choose leaner cuts like loin cuts and breast meat.

For total body wellness, aim to keep your saturated fat intake to less than 10 percent of your total calories.

Seafood is unique in that it gives you plenty of good-quality protein, as well as beneficial, heart-healthy fats like omega-3 fatty acids called docosahexae-noic acid (DHA) and eicosapentaenoic acid (EPA), which have been shown to keep your blood fats (lipids) like cholesterol and triglycerides in check. Plus, they have been linked to brain health and development, especially for infants and children, and may help to boost your mood and fend off depression. A recent review in the *Frontiers in Aging Neuroscience* reveals that low levels of EPA and DHA are linked to neurodegenerative disorders (especially DHA, because it has been shown to be the more beneficial for brain health).

Aim for at least 8 ounces of seafood per week to get the total body benefits. Fatty fish like salmon, tuna, sardines, anchovies, herring, and trout are good sources of omega-3 fats. The recommended total amount of EPA and DHA is 500 mg total per day, according to the Academy of Nutrition and Dietetics Position Paper: Dietary Fatty Acid for Healthy Adults. Avoid the high-mercury fish like shark, swordfish, tile fish, and king mackerel, especially for pregnant and breastfeeding women, and limit white tuna to 6 ounces per week.

The right protein balance

Ideally, for total body wellness, you should balance your protein sources so that you aren't just eating one type, but getting a mixture of good-quality lean sources. If you're vegetarian, alternate your plant proteins. If you're a meat-eater, mix in plants for a healthier, balanced approach.

Here's how to balance the proteins in your day. Aim to get 5½ to 6 ounces or protein per day:

✔ Scramble an egg for breakfast. Have a turkey sandwich (with 3 to 4 ounces of turkey) with lettuce and tomato for lunch. Sauté ½ cup tofu with vegetables for dinner.

✔ Toss 7 chopped walnut halves into a bowl of oatmeal for breakfast. Smear 2 tablespoons of hummus on a whole-grain wrap with vegetables for lunch. Grill 3 to 4 ounces of salmon with mixed vegetables for dinner.

✔ Toast whole-grain bread and spread with 1 tablespoon peanut butter for breakfast. Whip up a tuna salad (with 2 ounces of tuna) with diced cucumbers, shallots, and tomatoes for lunch. Bake a 3-ounce skinless chicken breast, and eat it with brown rice and broccoli for dinner.

An egg counts as one ounce of animal protein.

Fats

Eating fat in small amounts is essential because every cell in your body is made of fat (a lipid layer). Just keep in mind that fat is the most calorically dense nutrient. Fat contains 9 calories per gram, whereas carbs and protein contain 4 calories per gram. So measure out fats to control calories, but still get the health benefits!

What are the better fats for your total body wellness? Limit the saturated (solid) fat like butter, fatty cuts of beef or pork, dark meat of chicken or turkey, and high-fat dairy products like whole milk and full-fat cheese because saturated fat has been shown to increase risk for heart disease.

On the other hand, for heart-healthy fats, choose unsaturated (liquid) fats like vegetable oils, such as olive oil, canola oil, grapeseed oil, sunflower oil, safflower oil, and avocado oil. These oils contain both polyunsaturated and monounsaturated fats, which have proven beneficial for heart health and may help fend off inflammation in the body.

Oils

Vegetables oils have a health halo, but some are better than others as far as health properties. Steer clear of *partially hydrogenated vegetable oil,* which has hydrogen added to it to make it a solid, shelf-stable oil used in store-bought baked goods like cookies, cakes, muffins, and crackers. These foods most likely contain *trans fats,* which have been shown to pose a risk for heart disease because they've been shown to raise LDL (bad) cholesterol. Check the Nutrition Facts label and ingredients and avoid purchasing foods containing these types of oils and fats. Your heart will thank you with good health!

Cholesterol is *only* found in animal foods. Plant foods don't contain cholesterol. Although, cholesterol in foods may not affect your blood cholesterol levels, you'll get a lot of benefit from the unsaturated fat in plant foods like vegetable oils, avocado, nuts, and seeds. The Mediterranean diet containing these plant-based fats has been shown to be beneficial for fending off chronic disease like heart disease, type-2 diabetes, and high blood pressure, as well as inflammation.

Just because oil is good for you, doesn't mean you should dip bread liberally in olive oil at a restaurant or pour dressing over your mixed greens with reckless abandon. At 120 calories per tablespoon, oil should be drizzled cautiously and balanced with other fats into your daily meal plan to keep your waistline in check.

Table 5-5 shows how the calories add up in oils and foods that contain oils.

Table 5-5	Serving Sizes of Various Oils	
Oils	**Amount**	**Calories**
Vegetable oil (canola, corn, cottonseed, olive, peanut, safflower, soybean, sunflower)	1 tablespoon	120
Margarine, soft, without trans fats	1 tablespoon	100
Mayonnaise	1 tablespoon	100
Mayonnaise-type salad dressing	1 tablespoon	55
Italian dressing	2 tablespoons	85
Thousand Island dressing	2 tablespoons	120
Olives, canned	4 large	20
Avocado	½ medium	160
Peanut butter	1 tablespoon	190
Nuts (peanuts, mixed nuts, cashews, almonds, hazelnuts, sunflower seeds)	1 ounce	165 to 185

Source: www.choosemyplate.gov/food-groups/oils-counts.pdf

First-press extra-virgin olive oil is the least processed, anti-oxidant-rich variety. It's made from virgin (young) olives, which are known to have superior taste. The *first-press* part means that the olive was crushed only one time with a press. Plus, during processing the oil is not heated to over 80 degrees, which preserves its heart-healthy, monounsaturated fatty acids. Look for this on the label, as well as an opaque bottle to avoid light exposure. Store in a cool, dark place to prevent the oil from going rancid.

Nuts, seeds, and nut butters

Nuts are good food. Whether you prefer tree nuts (like almonds, pistachios, walnuts, cashews, or pecans) or legumes (like peanuts), they're a great source of unsaturated fats, monounsaturated fats, and polyunsaturated fats. Monounsaturated fats have been shown to decrease the detrimental LDL (bad) cholesterol and possibly raise the HDL (good) cholesterol. Polyunsaturated fats have been shown to be beneficial for overall health, especially brain health.

A recent study in the journal from the Public Library of Science, *PLOS One,* showed that eating tree nuts and/or peanuts is beneficial for decreasing risk for *metabolic syndrome,* a cluster of metabolic risk factors characterized by high blood sugar, abdominal fat, high blood pressure, and low HDL (good) cholesterol and high LDL (bad) cholesterol. All the more reason to eat nuts — plus, they taste good!

Table 5-6 shows how the nuts stack up for healthy fats.

Table 5-6	Amount of Fat in Various Nuts	
Nut (per Ounce)	*Polyunsaturated Fats (grams)*	*Monounsaturated Fats (grams)*
Almond nuts	3.5	9
Brazil nuts	7	7
Cashews	2	8
Hazelnuts	2	13
Macadamia nuts	0.5	17
Pecans	6	12
Pine nuts	10	5.5
Pistachios	4	7
Walnuts	13	2.5

Source: www.nuthealth.org

Walnuts are uniquely healthy nuts. They contain lots of polyunsaturated fat, including a plant-based omega-3 fat, alpha-linolenic acid (ALA). Seeds are also extremely healthy, offering beneficial omega-3 fats and ALA. For example, flaxseeds contain 1.6 grams of omega-3 fats per 1 ground tablespoon. (The fats in flaxseeds are better absorbed when the seed is ground versus whole.)

The recommended amount of ALA you should eat daily, according to the Academy of Nutrition and Dietetics position paper *Dietary Fatty Acids for Healthy Adults* is 1.1 grams a day for women and 1.6 grams per day for men. Flaxseeds are one of the most popular seeds for heart health. It's been studied extensively because the omega-3 fats in flaxseeds have been linked to heart health and may benefit cholesterol levels for the better.

Watch your portion sizes of nuts, nut butters, and seeds — they're high-calorie foods. Opt for varieties without added sugar and salt. Check the Nutrition Facts label for the serving size — a small amount every day goes a long way toward heart health and disease prevention. Store nut products in the refrigerator because the fats can go bad rapidly in the presence of heat and light.

Fatty fruits: Avocado and coconut

Believe it or not, fruit can contain fat, too! One of the most popular fatty fruits is avocado. Avocados contain a ton of heart-healthy monounsaturated fat and more potassium than bananas (which bodes well for your blood pressure). Plus, they're jam-packed with fiber, which can help fill you up longer, as well as help to keep your cholesterol levels in check and your intestines in good working order.

One-half of an avocado is 130 calories, so eating smaller amounts goes a long way. Here are some creative ways to get some healthy fat from avocado every day:

- ✔ Spread one-fifth of a ripe avocado on a whole-grain wrap, add veggies, and roll.
- ✔ Dice a slice of avocado over a mixed greens salad.
- ✔ Halve an avocado and fill each half with crab salad.
- ✔ Mash a whole avocado and mix in diced tomato, onion, cilantro, fresh lime juice, and a dash of salt for a tasty guacamole you can enjoy with friends.
- ✔ Puree avocado with berries and a dollop of plain yogurt for a tasty smoothie.

Another fruit with fat: coconut. Coconut is everywhere right now — from coconut flour to coconut milk to coconut water to coconut oil. This tropical fruit's fat is primarily saturated fat, which isn't good for you from a heart health standpoint.

Due to its fat composition, the Dietary Guidelines for Americans recommends that you limit saturated fat to less than 10 percent of your total calories. Eating coconut products is not currently recommended according to the Academy of Nutrition and Dietetics position paper *Dietary Fatty Acids for Healthy Adults.*

Knowing What to Keep in Check

As much as the Total Body Diet is about adding healthy foods into your life, there are some foods that you should limit. Foods that are highly processed with too much salt, added sugar, and solid fat should not be eaten regularly. In this section, I look at foods and ingredients that should be limited because they aren't doing your body any good or could be causing disease states to creep up.

Sugar

Sugar is in numerous foods and beverages. Naturally occurring sugars are found in milk products (from lactose) and fruits (from fructose), but the sugar that you want to be on the lookout for is sugar that's *added* during processing, preparation, or at the table. Sugars found naturally in foods are part of the food's total package of nutrients and other healthful components. Check ingredient lists on food labels for sugar added during processing as it can add up to extra calories.

Here are some common names that sugar goes by on food labels:

- Anhydrous dextrose
- Brown sugar
- Confectioner's powdered sugar
- Corn syrup
- Corn syrup solids
- Dextrin
- Fructose

- ✔ High-fructose corn syrup
- ✔ Honey
- ✔ Invert sugar
- ✔ Lactose
- ✔ Malt syrup
- ✔ Maltose
- ✔ Maple syrup
- ✔ Molasses
- ✔ Nectar
- ✔ Raw sugar
- ✔ Sucrose
- ✔ Sugar
- ✔ White granulated sugar

You aren't getting any nutritional value — just empty calories — from added sugar, so limit the candy, cookies, cakes, as well as sugary cereals, premarinated meats, and sugary beverages like smoothies, sugary sodas, gourmet coffee drinks, and lemonade.

Protein

Protein is the hot nutrient today. Just peruse the grocery store aisles and you'll see protein-fortified cereals, breads, pasta, juices, smoothies, and nutrition bars. But with all this protein, you could be overdoing it. Dairy products, as well as nuts, seeds, beans, and peas, contribute protein to the diet, too. If you get too much protein, it'll be stored as excess calories and may cause weight gain over time.

How do you know how much protein you should be eat every day? According to the Dietary Guidelines for Americans, in general, adults need between 46 and 56 grams of protein per day. You can track how much protein you're eating daily at www.supertracker.usda.gov.

Fat

Fat is important to get daily, especially the better-for-you fats — the unsaturated fat, monounsaturated fat, and polyunsaturated fat. Decreasing the saturated fat and replacing it with the better-for-you fat is a big bonus for decreasing heart disease risk. Keep in mind, though, that portion still counts — heart-healthy or not. A couple of tablespoons a day is all you need, so space them out throughout the day.

Watch for the liquid oils that are made solid through a process called hydrogenation. There are two types of hydrogenated oils: *fully hydrogenated oils*, which are firmer and do not contain unhealthy trans fats like the semi-soft, *partially hydrogenated oils*, used in shortening and soft margarine. Check food labels and avoid these fats as much as you can.

Salt

Salt is one of the world's oldest seasonings. Table salt is two minerals — sodium and chloride — which are needed to balance fluids (water) in the body. Sodium is an important mineral and electrolyte that is necessary for total body wellness. A little bit goes a long way, though!

Highly processed, packaged foods like baked goods, crackers, chips, cereals, and processed meats, such as salami, hot dogs, and bacon, are loaded with salt. Preparing foods yourself or looking for low-sodium or no-salt-added varieties can save you a lot of extra salt that your body does not need.

How much salt do you need every day? According to the Dietary Guidelines for Americans, the average adult, without high blood pressure, should aim to get no more than 2,300 mg of sodium per day. If you have high blood pressure or are at risk for it, are African American, have chronic kidney disease or diabetes, and are age 51 or older, drop your sodium intake to 1,500 mg per day.

Salt can add up fast, if you aren't watching it. Here's what a daily dose looks like :

- ✔ 2,300 mg of salt = 1 teaspoon
- ✔ 1,500 mg of salt = ⅔ teaspoon

A great way to decrease the salt, but increase flavor is to use herbs and spices. Plus, herbs and spices are salt-free, calorie-free, and offer a robust aromatic element. Look for salt-free seasoning blends, too. Here are some fun culinary tips for using herbs and spices in the kitchen:

- ✔ Toss fresh or dried basil and ginger into a vegetable omelet.
- ✔ Shake garlic powder (no garlic salt) into popped popcorn.

✔ Pop a sprig of fresh thyme into tomato soup or a chunky stew. Sprinkle dried thyme over pizza, scrambled eggs, or a tomato and cucumber salad.

✔ Sprinkle fresh rosemary leaves into diced sweet potatoes with extra-virgin olive oil, garlic, paprika and a dash of salt for a deliciously aromatic side dish.

✔ Stir a cinnamon stick into your coffee or hot chocolate. Sprinkle ground cinnamon over whole-grain toast and peanut butter.

Chapter 6

Focusing on Calories and Portion Size

· ·

In This Chapter

▶ Defining what a calorie is

▶ Determining your daily calorie needs

▶ Uncovering simple ways to manage calories

▶ Banishing overeating by becoming an expert portionist

· ·

Calories fuel your body every day for work, play, and rest, so it's important that you eat and drink good-quality calories so that you can function like a well-oiled machine. Good-quality calories come from foods like vegetables, fruits, whole grains, beans, legumes, nuts, seeds, loin cuts of beef and pork, fish, chicken and turkey breast, milk, cheese, and yogurt. On the other hand, sugar-laden calories from soft drinks, candy, cookies, cake, cereals, as well as fried chips, white-flour crackers, salty nut mixes, and fake-buttered popcorn, contain very little nutrition, so cutting back on these would do your body good.

Your total body health relies on a steady stream of good-quality calories. If you don't get that, health breakdowns can occur. According to the Centers for Disease Control and Prevention (CDC), poor nutrition is a leading cause of chronic diseases like diabetes, heart disease, stroke, obesity, and some cancers. So, understanding how and where to get good-quality fuel for your body is vital to ensuring optimal health for life!

In this chapter, you find out what calories are and why all calories are not created equal. You gain an understanding of how to manage your calories and how many calories you need to consume daily. Plus, you explore the world of servings versus portion sizes — and differentiate between the two once and for all. As you become an expert portionist, I also show you simple ways to be satisfied on fewer calories so you can put an end to overeating.

Getting the Inside Scoop on Calories

You don't have to look far or live long to hear about calories. Knowing how many calories you're eating at one time is helpful, but do you know what that number really means? When you have the calorie information in front of you, does it influence your decision on what to buy or eat? Knowing what the numbers *mean* is the key.

What are calories, anyway?

In science-speak, a *calorie* is a unit of energy. Calories actually provide your body with heat energy to allow your heart to beat, your brain to think, and your lungs to breathe. You can't function without calories. Getting enough calories to maintain the delicate balance of internal systems in your body is essential for survival.

Calories come in different types and have distinct forms and functions:

- **Carbohydrates:** Carbohydrates supply sugar (also known as glucose) to your cells for energy. Fruits, vegetables, breads, pasta, rice, milk, and yogurt all contain carbohydrates. Just as not all calories are created equal, not all carbs are created equal. Some carbs are higher in fiber and take longer to digest — which means they're better for your body. These better-for-you carbs are whole grains, vegetables, fruits, beans, peas, milk, and yogurt. Carbs that are high in refined sugar (like candy, cake, and cookies) lack nutritional value and should be consumed less often.

- **Proteins:** Proteins fuel and build your muscle mass and satisfy your appetite longer. Not all proteins are created equal. (Sensing a trend here?) High-quality protein sources include eggs, chicken and turkey breast, lean beef and pork (loin cuts), seafood, milk, cheese, yogurt, soymilk, tofu (soybean curd), seitan (wheat gluten), tempeh (fermented soybeans), and grains like quinoa and amaranth. More processed, fatty, and salty proteins — think bacon, salami, and sausage — should be eaten less often.

- **Fats:** Fats keep cell membranes intact, help your body absorb some nutrients, and make food taste good. Fats are vital to your health, but — as you probably guessed — some fats are better for you than others. The better-for-you fats are unsaturated, such as liquid vegetables oils like olive oil, grapeseed oil, and canola oil, as well as avocados, nuts (such as almonds, pistachios, and walnuts), seeds (such as flax, chia, and hemp), and cold-water, fatty fish like salmon, trout, halibut, tuna, mackerel, and cobia, which contain a type of polyunsaturated fat called omega-3 fatty acids, a heart-healthy fat. Saturated fats are solid at room temperature — like butter, bacon, cheese, cocoa butter (in milk chocolate), and coconut oil — and should be limited because they may contribute to heart disease.

Pregnant women, small children, and older adults should avoid large predatory fish like shark, swordfish, king mackerel, and tilefish because they're higher in mercury and other contaminants.

For total body wellness, the type of calories you take in should be balanced as follows:

- **Carbohydrate:** Roughly 45 percent to 65 percent of your daily calories should come from high-fiber carbs for sustained energy and to fuel your brain well over the course of the day. Choose less of the more-processed carbs.

- **Protein:** At least 10 percent and up to 35 percent of your daily calories should come from lean proteins from both plants and animals.

- **Fat:** Between 20 percent and 35 percent of your total calories can come from fat. Aim for mostly unsaturated fat. The saturated kind should be limited to no more than 7 percent to 10 percent of your total calories.

Figuring out your calorie needs for a day

How many calories you need is very different from what your next-door neighbor, child, or mother needs. Each of us has a unique calorie requirement based on gender, age, and amount of daily physical activity. Table 6-1 lists calorie requirements based on gender, age, and activity level.

Not sure what your activity level is? Here's a guide:

- **Sedentary:** A lifestyle that includes only the light physical activity associated with typical day-to-day life

- **Moderately active:** A lifestyle that includes physical activity equivalent to walking about 1½ to 3 miles per day at 3 to 4 miles per hour, in addition to the light physical activity associated with typical day-to-day life

- **Active:** A lifestyle that includes physical activity equivalent to walking more than 3 miles per day at 3 to 4 miles per hour, in addition to the light physical activity associated with typical day-to-day life

Managing calories in and out

The Total Body Diet is all about figuring out how to balance how many calories you eat with how many calories you expend through activity. When you know roughly how many calories you need to maintain your current weight or lose weight, you can tweak your intake accordingly.

Table 6-1		Calorie Requirements		
Gender	**Age**	**Sedentary**	**Moderately Active**	**Active**
Female	2–3 years	1,000 calories	1,000–1,400 calories	1,000–1,400 calories
	4–8 years	1,200 calories	1,400–1,600 calories	1,000–1,800 calories
	9–13 years	1,600 calories	1,600–2,000 calories	1,800–2,200 calories
	14–18 years	1,800 calories	2,000 calories	2,400 calories
	19–30 years	2,000 calories	2,000–2,200 calories	2,400 calories
	31–50 years	1,800 calories	2,000 calories	2,200 calories
	51 years and older	1,600 calories	1,800 calories	2,000–2,200 calories
Male	2–3 years	1,000 calories	1,000–1,400 calories	1,000–1,400 calories
	4–8 years	1,400 calories	1,400–1,600 calories	1,600–2,000 calories
	9–13 years	1,800 calories	1,800–2,000 calories	2,000–2,600 calories
	14–18 years	2,200 calories	2,400–2,800 calories	2,800–3,200 calories
	19–30 years	2,400 calories	2,600–2,800 calories	3,000 calories
	31–50 years	2,200 calories	2,400–2,600 calories	2,800–3,000 calories
	51 years and older	2,000 calories	2,200–2,400 calories	2,400–2,800 calories

Source: Dietary Guidelines for Americans, 2010

Think about your metabolism like a fire that you need to stoke frequently in order to keep it going. Now that you calculated your calorie needs (see the preceding section), you need to use those calories to your advantage and add activity throughout your day.

Do you feel hunger throughout the day? Do you know when you're full? One of the best ways to maintain a healthy body weight is to listen to your hunger and fullness cues. By becoming attuned to your appetite, you won't feel deprived and you'll eat only what your body needs. This process takes time and effort, so don't be frustrated with yourself if you don't get a handle on your appetite overnight. Just keep working at it every day, and view missteps as opportunities to learn about your body and what it needs.

Eating too many calories can cause your body to conserve calories as unused energy (in other words, store it as fat, which shows up as extra pounds on the scale or inches around your middle). But eating too few calories causes your metabolism to become sluggish. (Think of fire turning to embers in a fire pit.) Consuming the right amount of calories is a balancing act.

Here are some simple tips to balance calories in and out:

- ✔ Read food labels and know how many calories you're getting in a serving, to help track your calories in.

- ✔ Bring meals and snacks to work, school, or when you're out and about, so that you're mindful of the quantity and quality of what you're eating. Plus, you'll be prepared when hunger strikes and won't get the urge to eat convenient, less-nourishing food.

- ✔ Write down what you eat and drink right after you consume it. This way you won't forget what you ate, and you're less likely to overeat or skip meals. If you don't want to carry a notebook with you, use your smartphone! Chapter 16 lists a variety of smartphone apps, including several that are great for logging everything you eat and drink!

- ✔ Get regular physical activity to balance the calories you take in. By keeping your body and mind active, you use the calories you eat more efficiently.

- ✔ Keep your meals balanced with quality carbs, proteins, and healthy fats to satisfy your appetite longer and avoid cravings.

Becoming an Expert Portionist

Everywhere you go, portions are way too large. It's the get-your-money's-worth syndrome. At what cost, though? Your health pays the price because overindulging causes your blood sugar, blood pressure, and waistline to expand. So, becoming an expert *portionist* — someone who can eyeball a portion and know if it's the right size — is essential in a world where super-sizing runs rampant.

A large part of managing your daily calories is understanding the difference between a serving and a portion. A *serving* is a single standard unit of measure (used on a food label's Nutrition Facts label), and a *portion* is the amount you actually eat. For example, say you pick up a king-size candy bar when you're filling up your car's gas tank. If you check the Nutrition Facts label, you'll likely see that the candy bar has two servings — but if you're like most people, you eat the whole king-size candy bar, which is one portion. The average American eats more than one serving in a portion, which has a lot to do with our expanding waistlines.

Using smaller plates is a great way to keep your portions on the smaller side. Use appetizer plates for your regular meals. When you fill up a smaller plate or bowl, it gives you the illusion that you're eating a lot more than you actually are!

We eat with our eyes, as well as our stomachs, so when you see delicious-looking, abundant food on your plate, you feel satisfaction. However, nine times out of ten, your body doesn't need as much food as your eyes find appealing. Naturally, food excites our senses — and sight is one of them. But less can be more, if you think in terms of smaller cups, plates, and bowls.

Think and see smaller when it comes to food portions. Here are some simple ways to do that:

- ✔ **Measure it.** Get out your measuring cups, measuring spoons, and food scale. If you regularly scoop cereal or cooked rice, pasta, or quinoa into your measuring cup, you get to know pretty fast how much a cup is. You start to recognize a tablespoon of peanut butter or a 3-ounce piece of chicken breast.

- ✔ **Give it a hand.** Use your hand as a food measuring tool when measuring precisely isn't possible. The size of the palm of your hand is about 3 ounces of cooked meat, chicken, or fish. The tip of your thumb is a tablespoon of butter, and your fist is about a 1-cup serving. You might not carry your measuring cups and spoons with you to restaurants, but your hand is always with you!

- ✔ **Divide and conquer.** By divvying up your plate for whole grains, protein, vegetables, and fruits, you're more apt to stick with a reasonable portion and balance your meals better. Set aside one-quarter of the plate for grains, one-quarter for protein, and one-half for vegetables and fruits.

Putting the Halt on Calorie Overload

When you start eating, it can be challenging to stop, especially if the food tastes good. The exact causes of overeating vary from one person to the next, but regardless of your reason for overeating, there are ways to put a stop to it.

Eat like a bird, not a bear

One of the best ways to ensure that you don't overeat is to eat like a bird does. No, that doesn't mean living on worms and birdseed. Think about the way birds eat — they eat small beakfuls all day long as they flit around from place to place. With their high activity level, birds can't afford to be weighed down at any one meal. They're giving their bodies what they need at the moment and moving on.

Now, think about bears. They eat large amounts of food at one time to store up calories and gain fat to sustain themselves through their hibernation period. Most people don't need to store up calories and fat for later, so it's time to put an end to overloading on calories — unless you plan on going months without eating. (I didn't think so.)

A good rule of thumb is to fuel your body with small meals and snacks throughout the day so that your metabolism keeps humming along like a bird's does.

Check please! Leaving the table when you're done eating

If food is around, you'll eat it — at least if you're like most people. According to *Mindless Eating: Why We Eat More Than We Think,* by Brian Wansink, PhD (Bantam), we have an imperfect food memory, especially when dining out. One of his studies revealed that five minutes after leaving an Italian restaurant, 31 percent of people couldn't remember how much bread they ate and 12 percent of the bread eaters denied having any bread at all!

Avoid getting lulled into overeating when eating out by doing the following:

- Eat slowly by putting your utensils down between bites.
- Nix the appetizers. Order your entree right away.
- Ask for the bread, butter, chips, and dip to be removed from the table.
- Downsize your plates by ordering small appetizer sizes or half-orders.
- Share your meals and desserts.
- Doggy-bag half of your meal before you eat.
- Set a limit on what you want to spend. Then you'll stick with a lower-calorie budget, too!

Banishing the nighttime cravings

What is it about the evenings that bring on cravings? Well, for one thing, if you work a standard 9-to-5 job, your work is done — at least for the next 8 to 12 hours — so you can relax. Along with relaxation comes feelings of wanting to eat something — and typically that something is salty, fatty, or sugary. (Most people don't get late-night cravings for a piece of fruit.) You fall into your easy chair when you get home and grab a pint of ice cream or a bag of your favorite chips and mindlessly munch away the stress of your day!

It's not that you can't eat at night — it's what and how much you're eating. First, stop eating at least two hours before bedtime — if you hit the hay at 11 p.m., stop eating by 9 p.m. This way, you give your body time to digest your food properly and you don't go to bed on a full stomach. If you want an evening snack after dinner, be sure it contains some form of protein to stabilize your blood sugar and control your appetite. Finally, take one serving in a small bowl or plate and enjoy it — never eat out of a bag, carton, container, or box (unless it's a single serving size).

Revamp your evening eating with the following Total Body Diet–approved snack suggestions:

- ✔ 1 tablespoon nut butter plus one small piece of fruit (sliced) on a large plain rice cake

- ✔ 1 tablespoon ground flax seed or chia or hemp seed plus 1 tablespoon dried fruit mixed into a cup of plain Greek yogurt

- ✔ A serving of fruit plus ½ cup lowfat cottage cheese

- ✔ 2 tablespoons hummus and sliced veggies in a small whole-grain pita

- ✔ Six whole-grain crackers and ½ cup plain Greek yogurt with a drizzle of honey

- ✔ ½ ounce of nuts and a small piece of fruit

- ✔ 3 cups of popped popcorn sprinkled with grated parmesan and garlic powder

Nighttime eating doesn't have to ruin your whole day. If you have a hankering to eat after dinner, be sure to keep it portion controlled and balanced with protein and a healthy carbohydrate. You'll see cravings disappear as you create a new nighttime eating regimen. Many times thirst is masked as hunger, so drink a glass of water when you feel hungry and check in 30 minutes later to see if you're still feeling hungry for food.

Chapter 7

Move, Move, Move: Understanding the Importance of Exercise

. . . .

In This Chapter

▶ Gearing up for total body rewards above and beyond your fitness dreams

▶ Discovering why everyday movement matters

▶ Fitting fitness into your daily routine

. . . .

*F*itness and health go hand in hand. Just as healthy eating matters to your total body wellness, so does moving every day. Keeping fit and active helps get your muscles, brain, and metabolism going. No matter what type of activity you enjoy, moving your body is beneficial.

Before diving into this chapter, gauge your fitness efforts by asking yourself some questions:

✔ Do you try to get up from your desk by standing or walking at least once every hour?

✔ Do you take the stairs instead of the elevator?

✔ Do you aim for at least 30 minutes of activity five days a week?

✔ Do you stretch at least once a day?

✔ Do you park farther away from stores or your office building to walk more?

✔ Do you mix up your activity with aerobic activity (walking, jogging, swimming, and so on) with muscle-strengthening exercises (such as yoga, Pilates, sit-ups, pushups, and weight lifting)?

If you answered "yes" to the majority of these questions, you're already doing great! If you answered "no," don't fret! This is the perfect time to make lifestyle changes to enhance your total body wellness. And this chapter shows you how.

Reaping the Rewards of Fitness

According to the President's Council on Physical Fitness, *fitness* is a measure of the body's ability to function efficiently and effectively in work and leisure times, to be healthy, to resist *hypokinetic diseases* (diseases that stem from a sedentary lifestyle), and to meet emergency situations.

The rewards of physical fitness are immense. And every year, scientists learn new ways that fitness positively impacts human health. The science shows that regular movement can help you

- ✔ Maintain your flexibility, muscle and bone strength (which are vital as you get older), and posture
- ✔ Keep a brighter, sunnier outlook
- ✔ Maintain clearer, sharper thinking during the day
- ✔ Sleep more soundly at night

In this section, I focus more on each of these benefits of physical fitness.

Maintaining flexibility, strength, and posture

Fitness gives your total body a boost! Not only does it keep your heart and brain functioning well, but it also keeps your body flexible and standing strong. As you move through life, fitness makes regular activities like tying your shoes, putting on your socks, and maintaining good form and posture possible. Fitness is not only about weight loss and maintenance (although that's a large part of it); it's also about gaining muscles or lean body mass, which burns more calories at rest than fat mass does — a big bonus! From core strength to maintaining strength and flexibility through your body, a good fitness regimen allows you to function at a higher level and decreases the risk of falls and injury with age.

Elevating your mood

One of the best benefits of physical fitness is that it enhances mental fitness, too. You can fend off the blues and possibly reduce the risk of depression by getting up and moving. Movement is an essential part of life. If your body doesn't get activity every day, your total body — including your mind — suffers the consequences. On the upside, an active lifestyle can help improve your mood.

Just getting in the pool or hitting the road walking can keep your mood in good working order. The science on exercise and mental health has shown that regular activity brings with it a sense of physical, as well as psychological, well-being. Exercise causes changes in your brain. It releases serotonin and dopamine — two chemicals that bathe your brain with good feelings and make you want to do that behavior again. Physical activity has been shown to alleviate symptoms of depression because it activates changes in your brain's main control tower (the central nervous system).

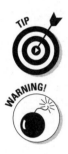

Keep a mood and activity log. It'll help you see which activities make you feel better mentally and physically. Note your mood before and after engaging in a specific activity.

Mood disorders are a group of distinct disturbances in a person's mood or behavior, which include *major depression* (symptoms of which include chronic sadness, feelings of hopelessness, appetite loss, or overeating), *bipolar disorder* (characterized by swings of bliss and depression), and *anxiety disorder* (a group of emotional disturbances characterized by fear and chronic worrying). If you think you have one of these disorders, consult with your healthcare provider to set a care plan in place. Don't try to rely on exercise to boost your mood instead of going to a medical professional for help. Exercise can do great things for mood, but it can't cure mental health disorders.

Thinking crystal clear

A big bonus of exercise is that it can clear out mental cobwebs. When you exercise regularly, you think more clearly, have more creativity, and are more productive throughout the day. If you want to get a mental task done well, "walk on it" (go for a walk and think it over). With activity, your blood will flow to your brain, releasing all sorts of new and creative ways to tackle a problem, offer solutions, and come up with a new and exciting plan of attack.

Exercise has been shown to boost energy to the brain and increase mental output, boosting productivity. Plus, exercise can elevate mood — and a happier you is a more productive you!

According to the Physical Activity Guidelines for Americans, there is strong evidence to support that regular physical activity can cause better mental function in older adults. So get your body and mind moving today!

The potential benefits of exercise — especially aerobic activity that gets your heart and blood pumping — on the brain are amazing. It may help improve memory, may enable you to focus more clearly, and may even fend off dementia.

Getting a good night's sleep

Sleep is vital to good health. To help fend off a number of health problems (including mood disorders, obesity, high blood pressure, and high blood sugar), as well as help your body in the repair and recovery of all your organs, aim for at least seven hours of sleep per night. Here's the good news: Exercise can be a natural sleep aid. In fact, it's among the National Sleep Foundation's recommendations for getting a good night's sleep.

If you aren't sleeping well or you want to determine the quality of your sleep, keep a sleep diary. There are monitors and smartphone apps to determine how much sleep you're getting. Check out www.sleepfoundation.org for tools and tips to getting a good night's sleep, but here are some tips to get you started:

- ✔ **Stick to a sleep schedule.** Go to bed and wake up at the same time every day, whether it's a workday or the weekend.

- ✔ **Practice a relaxing bedtime ritual.** That might mean taking a bath or reading a good book. Wind down an hour before going to sleep.

- ✔ **Avoid late afternoon naps.** They may inhibit nighttime sleep.

- ✔ **Keep your room cool.** Somewhere between 60 and 67 degrees is typically best for sleep.

- ✔ **Get a comfortable mattress and pillows.** An old, uncomfortable mattress won't do you much good. Take the time to shop for a mattress that suits your needs.

- ✔ **Avoid bright lights in your bedroom at night.** This includes your cellphone and laptop. Staring at the blue light of an electronic screen can make it hard to fall asleep at night.

- ✔ **Avoid alcohol, cigarettes, and heavy meals in the evening.**

- ✔ **Keep your work out of your bedroom.** Don't lie in bed with your laptop, phone, or paperwork.

- ✔ **Keep a detailed sleep diary.** You can find a useful one at www.sleepfoundation.org/sleep-diary/SleepDiaryv6.pdf.

Consistency is key

The best way to reap the total body rewards of fitness is to be consistent with your efforts. If you only have time for a short walk or stretch on Monday, bounce back the next day with a longer walk or run, along with a good cooldown and stretch.

One day does not dictate your fitness level just as one food does not make or break your waistline. Be realistic and forgiving with yourself to design a fitness routine that is empowering, sustainable over the long term, and diverse enough to fend off boredom. Find indoor and outdoor activities that you enjoy so that weather doesn't keep you from moving.

How do you stay consistent with your exercise routine? Think about the carrot that is dangling in front of you — in other words, the reward that being fit offers. The reward of fitness is unique to you. Whether it's simply being able to fit into your favorite jeans or having more energy during the day or toning and strengthening your body to make everyday tasks simple or knowing that you're keeping your blood pressure, cholesterol, and blood sugar in check, focus on that benefit. If you do, you'll make exercise a part of your daily life — and soon it'll be a good habit that's hard to break.

WARNING! If your sleep is disrupted due to pauses in your breathing while you sleep, you could have a sleep disorder called *sleep apnea*, which can be serious. Consult your healthcare provider or a sleep professional for assistance.

Making Small Changes in Your Daily Life

Lots of people get overwhelmed at the thought of exercise. They envision themselves having to hang out in gyms with beefy bodybuilder types, and they let that stop them from doing anything at all. But it doesn't have to take a lot of time to become more active and learn to make good moves in your life. Think about it: You can do leg lifts as you wash dishes or shoulder rolls as you're driving your kids around town. Even mundane tasks in life can offer an opportunity to use your muscles and gain strength in areas that you never thought possible!

Take a look at the following chart and see how you can make somewhat sedentary activities more active.

Activity	How to Make It More Active
Reading a book	Hop on an elliptical machine or treadmill and read while you exercise.
Computer work	Get a standing desk to alternate sitting and standing.
Folding laundry	As you fold laundry, do side or back leg lifts (alternate lifting each leg to the side and back, ten times per side).
Talking on the phone	While you talk, do squats or wall presses (put your back against a wall, lower your body to a seated position, and hold for ten seconds).
Watching TV	Do sit-ups, do push-ups, or lift weights while you watch. If you're afraid of missing all the action, leave the exercise for the commercial breaks.

You don't have to go to a gym to get a proper work out. A large part of the Total Body Diet is making fitness part of your everyday life. By bending, stretching, and walking daily, you're doing your body good.

How can you do more for your body every day? Take a ten-minute break from your daily activities at least three times a day. That'll add up to the 30 minutes of activity you need. Not sure what you can possibly accomplish in ten minutes? Here are some ideas:

- ✔ Water your plants or take the garbage out.

- ✔ Walk around your block as fast as you can.

- ✔ Get on the floor or a yoga mat and stretch. If you can't get on the floor at work, sit up straight at your desk and stretch your arms up to the ceiling, turn your head from side to side, touch your chin to your chest, and roll your neck gently. Repeat three times, breathing in and out with purpose.

- ✔ Walk up and down the stairs to get your blood pumping and leg muscles working.

In the practice of yoga, moving (and living) with *intention,* or a goal in mind, is a powerful player in transforming your life. If you make a mental intention to move more, your body will follow. Let your intentions lead you to the next activity, and pretty soon moving more will become a natural part of your life. Just as planning your meals and snacks brings purpose to your daily routine, so will mindful movement. Set a realistic weekly goal, and as you progress, add another day or two to your schedule until you're getting 30 minutes of activity a day at least five days a week.

Standing room only is ideal

You may pay less for standing-room-only tickets at a concert, but in the long run, you're getting more for your money because standing is ideal for your health. Humans are made to stand upright — not sit for too long. Our modern, computer age tends to encourage a sedentary lifestyle. In fact, some office workers sit for as much as 15 hours a day!

Science is delving into solutions to this global issue of how sitting affects human health. Recent research in the journal *Diabetologica* shows that sitting too much may be a risk factor for multiple chronic diseases, such as obesity, type-2 diabetes, cardiovascular disease, multiple types of cancer, bone disease, and sexual dysfunction. As a result, a sedentary lifestyle causes healthcare costs to soar.

The good news is, you can take charge of your health and help reduce the risk of diseases associated with sitting too much in the following ways:

- ✔ If you work in an office, get a sit-stand desk that adjusts so that you can have increments of sitting broken up with standing.
- ✔ Get up and walk during conference calls, if possible.
- ✔ Climb the stairs throughout the day.
- ✔ Take a walking lunch break.
- ✔ Walk to and from the train or bus stop.
- ✔ Walk to the grocery store.
- ✔ Skip the drive-thru bank and walk in to do your banking instead.
- ✔ Bike, walk, or rollerblade to and from work.

Move More, Weigh Less

It makes sense that the more your move, the more fit you'll be. But it's not that simple — activity alone doesn't keep your weight in a healthy range. You have to think about how much you're eating and not eat more than you're burning — whether you're active or not.

The first step is to know how much you're burning just by being alive — that's called your *basal metabolic rate* (BMR). You can calculate your BMR by entering your weight, height, age, and gender in an online calculator (for example, the one at `www.myfitnesspal.com/tools/bmr-calculator` — or just search the web for "BMR calculator"). Your BMR tells you how much you would burn if you rested 24/7.

Beyond your BMR, you burn calories doing daily activities (for example, getting dressed, brushing your teeth, walking around your house, going out to get the mail, and so on). And you also burn calories through exercise. The number of calories you burn doing activities depends on how much you weigh — the more you weigh, the more calories you burn.

Table 7-1 shows how many calories are burned by a 154-pound man in a variety of activities. Odds are, you aren't a 154-pound man, but these numbers just give you a sense of how many calories you can burn doing different activities.

Table 7-1	Calories Burned by a 154-Pound Man
Physical Activity	*Calories Burned in 30 Minutes*
Running/jogging (5 mph)	295
Bicycling (more than 10 mph)	295
Swimming (slow freestyle laps)	255
Aerobics	240
Walking (4.5 mph)	230
Heavy yard work (chopping wood)	220
Weight lifting (vigorous effort)	220
Basketball (vigorous)	220
Hiking	185
Light gardening/yard work	165
Dancing	165
Golf (walking and carrying clubs)	165
Bicycling (less than 10 mph)	145
Walking (3.5 mph)	140
Weight training (general light workout)	110
Stretching	90

*Source: ChooseMyPlate.gov (*www.choosemyplate.gov/physical-activity/ calories-burn.html*)*

If you don't want to have to do a bunch of math, calculating your BMR and exactly how many calories you burned while doing the tango, you might want to take advantage of technology. A variety of websites — for example, Lose It! (www.loseit.com) and myfitnesspal (www.myfitnesspal.com) — allow you to track your weight, food, and exercise and tell you, how many calories you can eat per day and reach your weight loss goal (or maintain your current weight if you're where you want to be).

Losing the scale and focusing on action

The best thing you can do for your total body wellness is to stop relying on the numbers on your bathroom scale. Create a different scale of possibilities for yourself! If you're living an active lifestyle and eating well, focus on setting new fitness goals. Ask yourself the following questions:

✔ Do you feel good about your activity today? Why or why not?

✔ Did you move more than yesterday? Why or why not?

✔ What could you do differently tomorrow?

✔ What new activities would you like to try this week or month?

Walking your way toward health

Whether you're a seasoned fitness buff or a newbie to the world of physical fitness, counting steps with a pedometer — whether on a wrist band, waist clip, or even your smartphone — has become a popular way to track individual physical fitness. Having a goal — a number of steps you're aiming to get in every day — is important. The Physical Activity Guidelines for Americans (PAG) has a great road map to setting your step goals. Here's one way to set your own step goal:

1. **Determine your usual daily steps from your baseline activity.**

   Wear or carry a pedometer to observe the number of steps you take on several ordinary days with no episodes of walking for exercise, and calculate the average. Let's say you walk 3,500 steps on Sunday, 5,500 steps on Monday, and 6,000 steps on Tuesday. Do the math: 3,500 + 5,500 + 6,000 = 15,000 steps ÷ 3 days = 5,000 steps per day on average.

2. **Determine how many steps you take during ten minutes of an exercise walk.**

   Wear or carry the pedometer, and measure the number of steps you take. For the sake of this example, let's say you come up with 1,000 steps in ten minutes. For a goal of 30 minutes of walking for exercise, your total number of steps would be 1,000 × 3 = 3,000 steps. (The number of minutes you walk for exercise in a given day is up to you, but 30 minutes per day is a great goal to start with. *Remember:* You don't have to do one 30-minute walk. Break it up into two or three shorter walks if that works better for you.)

3. **Calculate your daily step goal.**

   Add your average daily steps from Step 1 to the number of steps required for a 30-minute walk (3,000), to get the total steps per day: 5,000 + 3,000 = 8,000 steps.

This is a great goal to start with. When you start counting your steps, you may find yourself intentionally parking farther away from buildings just to get a few more steps in. For many people, counting steps can become a fun game — a way to see if they can top themselves by walking a little more than they did the day before!

Chapter 8

Assembling Your Total Body Diet Team

"No man (or woman) is an island; entire of itself."

—John Donne, poet

You are not alone in your journey toward total body wellness. Dialing into your health needs involves embracing the value of a support system around you. Whether you're carving out new lifestyle changes or reinforcing healthy lifestyle changes that you've made already, developing a supportive environment goes a long way. You may look at people who have been successful with weight loss or maintenance and wonder, how do they do it? Many times there's a lot of behind-the-scenes work, such as social and online support, professional guidance, and group meetings.

According to the American Psychological Association, sticking with a weight loss plan is easier when you have support, share tips on diet and exercise, and have an exercise buddy. A study in the *International Journal of Behavioral Medicine,* which looked at the factors to weight loss maintenance after a two-year weight loss diet program among 12 women (54 to 71 years old), revealed through interviews with the participants that clear personal goals and support from family and friends seem to be of major importance for long-term maintenance of new dietary habits. Relationships inside the home as spouse support, according to this research, was a big factor in maintaining weight loss goals.

In this chapter, I take a deep dive into the numerous ways to access support for your total body wellness goals.

These support techniques and tools can be used together or separately. There are no right or wrong ways to go. Support systems are dynamic players in your continual journey toward total body health and wellness. Experimenting with what works for you is the best bet. You may find group support beneficial at one point, but then turn to one-on-one counseling as your go-to method of support. Do what works for you — and if one method is not working, try another.

Understanding the Importance of a Support Team

Your need for support is unique to you. Before you leap into assembling a team, consider some ways that support teams — which can include many different people like family, friends, co-workers, as well as healthcare professionals — can benefit you. Support teams can

- ✔ Offer guidance and new resources, tips, and tools
- ✔ Be a sounding board to overcome obstacles and setbacks
- ✔ Point out areas of progress (because it's sometimes hard to see it yourself!)
- ✔ Create new connections for you by providing a new community
- ✔ Foster growth and confidence (as you push past your comfort zone)
- ✔ Help you to create realistic expectations for growth and change
- ✔ Motivate you when boredom or fatigue sets in

Now that you know what a support team can do for you. Let's look at ways to find one that fits with your personality and lifestyle needs.

Assembling a good healthcare team

Part of your support group can begin with your healthcare team, which can start as one healthcare professional. For example, your initial support can begin with a registered dietitian nutritionist (RDN) who can offer you support with making healthful food choices and meal planning. The RDN can then make referrals to other appropriate professionals as needed, such as:

- ✔ **Physician/physician's assistant:** Can offer medical support and answer questions based on overall health and disease prevention and management

- ✔ **Nurse/nurse practitioner:** Can offer medical support and guidance for disease prevention and management

- ✔ **Psychologist/counselor:** Can offer psychological support through therapy, which includes skill building, goal setting, and work to do at home

- ✔ **Personal trainer/exercise physiologist:** Can offer exercise support with individualized physical activities that can fit into your lifestyle and assist with disease management and prevention

When a variety of healthcare professionals work together offering their unique skills and expertise, that's called an *interdisciplinary team* approach. If you're working with more than one healthcare professional at a time, there should be open communication among all of you. Each of the healthcare providers should feel free to call, email, or meet with the others to discuss your work together. This establishes continuity of care and keeps everyone on the same page!

What to look for in a nutrition expert

A registered dietitian (RD) *is* a nutritionist, but a nutritionist is *not* necessarily a registered dietitian. When looking for a food and nutrition expert, look for the letters RD or RDN after the person's name. When you see those letter, you have the added assurance that the person has

- ✔ **Received nutrition education and training from an accredited dietetics program and passed a competitive registration exam.** A bonus is that about half of the RDs and RDNs hold graduate degrees and many have certificates in specialized fields like weight management, sports, culinary, pediatric, renal, oncology, or gerontological nutrition.

- ✔ **Completed a dietetics internship.** An internship is 900 hours of supervised practice in multiple areas of the nutrition field, including a healthcare facility, foodservice operation, and community agency.

- ✔ **Continued to foster learning through continuing professional education units (CPEUs).** At least 75 CPEUs must be completed every five years to maintain the RD/RDN credential.

- ✔ **Tailored individualized nutrition programs.** These programs offer creative, out-of-the-box meal plans, grocery shopping, and culinary tips, as well as food journaling and mindful eating strategies.

Part of finding the right healthcare team is knowing what the best fit is for you. Support teams come in many different packages and all these professionals may not be necessary. It's good to know what types of professionals are available, but don't forget that family and friends can offer vital support, too!

Shopping around

Every healthcare professional comes at their work in a unique way and you want to be sure that it's in agreement with your philosophy from the beginning. Finding a healthcare professional is a bit like dating — not everyone is right for you!

Here are some questions to ask during your initial meeting with your healthcare provider:

- ✔ **How often do you want to follow up with me?**
- ✔ **Can I ask you questions via email as they come up, or would you prefer I save them for face-to-face visits?**
- ✔ **How many sessions do you require with a typical patient?**
- ✔ **How do you assess progress in your patients?**
- ✔ **Do you accept insurance for services?** Under the Affordable Care Act, certain preventive services are covered, such as diet counseling for those at high risk for chronic diseases. For a complete list, visit www.healthcare.gov/preventive-care-benefits.
- ✔ **What is your cancellation policy?** There is typically a fee for service if someone cancels within 24 hours.
- ✔ **Will we set goals together at every session?**
- ✔ **Do you allow your patients to take the lead or do you prefer to?**

How do you even know where to begin to find healthcare professionals to comprise your Total Body Diet team? There are a number of ways to go about shopping around for a support team. Here are some options:

- ✔ **Ask your current healthcare provider for recommendations.** Whether you're asking your doctor for a referral to a clinical psychologist or an RDN, use your current healthcare provider as a multidisciplinary springboard. Primary care doctors are a great resource because they have access to a plethora of providers locally and nationally.

✔ **Inquire at your local hospital.** Hospitals offer in-patient services, as well as outpatient services for people seeking assistance who do not need to be admitted to the hospital. Hospitals also have community relations specialists who organize a plethora of support programs to assist with all facets of healthcare needs and can link you up with departments and provider referrals.

✔ **Contact your local chamber of commerce.** They can assist you with finding local experts in your area. Many expert groups hold monthly roundtable discussion on various health topics for the public to attend. This is an easy and comfortable way to mix and mingle with more than one healthcare provider at a time and gain connections in your community.

✔ **Ask your local grocery store if there's a registered dietitian nutritionist (RDN) on staff.** Many supermarkets employ RDNs as part of their team inside the store to point out better products to the customers, highlight recipe ideas, and offer one-on-one nutrition counseling to answer individual questions pertaining to food choices, meal planning, and overall health.

✔ **Ask your friends and family for referrals.** If you feel comfortable inquiring within the close network of people around you, that's a viable way to find support and assistance. Plus, the people who know you best may be more apt to steer you toward someone who is well suited for you.

✔ **Use an online referral service.** A myriad of web pages are devoted to finding healthcare professionals from every discipline. For example, to locate a local RDN that specializes in what you need, go to the Find an Expert page at www.eatright.org. You simply search in your area and contact names will come up — it's that simple.

Don't get discouraged if right off the bat you aren't in sync with your healthcare professional. It takes time to develop a working relationship based on mutual trust, respectful communication, and give and take. One or two meetings don't make or break your success with your support team member. It's important to give it a little time and learn to lean on your team before you begin.

Leaning on your team

When you get a couple healthcare members on your team, you can begin to build a relationship with them. Just as with any partnership, a healthy relationship is a priority to your happiness and success. At first, you may want to forge ahead on your own, but over time you may realize that learning to lean on a team of professionals, friends, and family members is a safety net that gives you the security that you can quickly recover from minor setbacks.

For a quick way to think about how to LEAN on your support team, think of it this way:

- ✔ **L**et someone know about your successes and setbacks this week.
- ✔ **E**volve with gradual communication. A small interaction goes a long way.
- ✔ **A**ctively seek out support and don't wait for it to come to you.
- ✔ **N**avigate your own path to success by listening and taking recommendations at your discretion.

At first you may have a hard time trusting and revealing your daily doings about your eating and exercise to your support team, but over time you'll see the value of asking for guidance and help if you feel like you aren't on the right path. **_Remember:_** Support runs the gamut from a quick check-in email to a phone call to a face-to-face meeting. Whatever you see fit as support, that's what will work for you.

Ask yourself some questions after your interactions with your support team:

- ✔ Do I feel encouraged?
- ✔ Are our interactions constructive and do they move me to make and maintain positive changes?
- ✔ Am I learning anything about myself?
- ✔ Do I want to meet or communicate more or less frequently?
- ✔ Are there ways that I can better utilize my support team?

If you aren't happy with the support you're receiving, there is nothing wrong with politely moving on to another provider. If the connection isn't there, it's not there. Here are some signs that it may be time to call it quits with a member of your support team:

- ✔ **One-way communication:** You don't get return emails or phone calls in a timely manner.
- ✔ **Brief interactions:** The responses you get are short and don't offer much information.
- ✔ **Lack of enthusiasm:** Meetings aren't positive and encouraging.
- ✔ **Chronic rescheduling:** The team member makes frequent last-minute cancellations.

The Total Body Diet mentality is as much about what you eat and drink as it is about how you gain a sense of responsibility for taking charge of your health with your choices, actions, and the support you gain along the way. With small steps and the will to keep moving forward regardless of the obstacles, you'll feel more fulfilled, moving through life with a sense of ownership toward your own health and happiness.

Looking at Your Support Options

Support comes in a variety of ways these days. You can find

- ✔ Solo support with one-on-one counseling
- ✔ Group meetings with interactive discussions
- ✔ Online support with food diaries and photos and professional feedback

There are pros and cons of each. There is no one-size-fits-all solution and you may find that what works at one point in your goal setting may not work at another. You can also do these methods together — attend group meetings, seek out one-on-one support, and track foods with a smartphone app at the same time. In this section, I fill you in on the pros and cons of each type of support system.

Support groups: Becoming a groupie

Since the beginning of time, men and women have met in support-type groups to discuss family news and the world around them. Dan Buettner, author and longevity expert, talks about the most primitive of support groups in his book, *The Blue Zones: 9 Lessons for Living Longer.* For example, Buettner found that the women of Okinawa who live to 100+ years old meet every day for tea time discussions about the news of the day and to support each other's lives with laughter, love, and healthy gossip. They offer same gender support and Buettner counts this as longevity therapy for these centenarians. It's the same with modern-day book groups, bible study groups, and sports enthusiast groups — they offer support for a common purpose.

For Total Body Diet enthusiasts, group support can have pluses and minuses. Here are some of the most common advantages of support groups:

- ✔ They generate creative eating solutions and recipe ideas.
- ✔ They offer meal-planning tips.

- ✔ They can help you brainstorm exercise strategies.
- ✔ They foster creativity and exchange of thoughts and ideas.
- ✔ They offer a sense of community.

Nothing is perfect, and support groups are no exception. Here are some drawbacks to meeting with support groups:

- ✔ You can be given inaccurate information and unhealthy dieting practices by group members.
- ✔ Dominant members can lead the group off track.
- ✔ One person's negative thinking can spread through the whole group.
- ✔ Quieter participants may not feel comfortable revealing their thoughts.
- ✔ Personality conflicts can occur among group members.
- ✔ Meeting times may not be convenient.

A good facilitator can help keep the group heading in the right direction with all members keeping their individual goals in mind — without getting side-tracked and causing members to lose interest. The positive nature of the group should always be a priority.

Finding support online

People are more reliant on computers and computer technology than ever before. A review in the *Journal of Diabetes Science and Technology* showed that the use of tech tools can result in improved long-term weight management and cost-effectiveness by allowing

- ✔ Treatment recommendations to be delivered to individuals remotely
- ✔ More opportunities for self-monitoring and tracking health-related data
- ✔ Widespread and speedy dissemination of health information and recommendations
- ✔ Increased patient-dietitian/physician contact

A more recent review in the American Heart Association's journal, *Circulation*, examined mobile health technologies in the prevention of cardiovascular disease. It revealed that although more research is needed in determining how mobile devices can aid in creating lasting lifestyle changes, there's big potential in this arena. Mobile health technologies are seen as an important adjunct to face-to-face appointments and counseling because information can be shared more rapidly and target individual behavior change. In addition, mobile health allows patients to record blood pressure and blood sugar readings in their natural settings, which can contribute to greater accuracy. Therefore, researchers encourage the use of new technologies in conjunction with traditional healthcare to generate more evidence of its effectiveness over the long haul.

All you have to do is sit down at your computer or with your smartphone, and you have access to a support system. With an estimated 63 percent of Americans having access to the Internet by way of a smartphone, according to a recent research by Pew Internet, web-based applications for delivery via mobile devices are at the forefront of many health conditions, including diabetes, overweight/obesity, mental health, tobacco use, and many others. Now you can track your food and beverage intake very easily with a variety of online apps and websites, such as www.supertracker.usda.gov.

Many people like the convenience and comfort of support online, whether with groups or individual one-on-one counseling. With numerous programs available — from apps to websites to chat rooms devoted to health and wellness — this is a viable option for a broad spectrum of age groups and health needs. In fact, researchers are suggesting that that next era of weight management will design virtual clinics, in which data will be transmitted from individuals remotely in their home to the healthcare team.

Using apps to track dietary intake instead of using traditional pen and paper, people lost significantly more weight, according to a pilot randomized control trial in the *Journal of Medical Internet Research.* For more about online tools and apps, check out Chapter 16.

Some of the benefits of support online include the following:

- ✔ It saves time with no travel.
- ✔ It's less expensive than traditional methods.
- ✔ You can participate from anywhere.
- ✔ It may not be as intimidating as face-to-face meetings.
- ✔ You can track your own dietary intake and physical activity.

On the other hand, support online can have drawbacks, such as the following:

- ✔ You need a smartphone or computer with Internet access.
- ✔ Technology can be intimidating, if you don't know how to use it.
- ✔ Support isn't as intimate when you're in front of a screen instead of face to face.

> ✔ You may not be as invested emotionally without interacting with other people in person.
>
> ✔ It's easy to get sidetracked and miss online meetings.
>
> ✔ User burnout causes dropout.

Whether used alone or as support to a more intensive intervention, web-based apps and tracking tools have shown to be successful. They have universal applications because they can be isolated to an individual, encourage family participation, or be connected to a larger social network.

According to *Circulation,* for weight management there are a number of mobile methods, such as texting, smartphone apps, handheld personal digital assistants (PDAs), interactive voice response (IVR) systems, and e-scales and wireless physical activity monitoring devices (like the FitBit and JawBone). The evidence shows the greatest weight loss success is achieved with comprehensive, multicomponent programs that are personally tailored, promote regular self-monitoring, and involve a qualified professional to provide the intervention. In other words, web-based care should be integrated into traditional care plans to increase treatment effectiveness (weight loss and permanent lifestyle changes).

One-on-one counseling

The most intimate of all the support methods, one-on-one counseling allows for an exchange of ideas, thoughts, and feelings. With personalized recommendations, this form of support allows for interpersonal communication between you and your healthcare provider. There may even be a contractual agreement, whether written or spoken, that sets the goals of the working relationship. The contract cements the expectations for the meetings, creating an ongoing set of boundaries.

Some of the benefits of one-on-one counseling can be the following:

> ✔ There's a greater sense of accountability when meeting face to face.
>
> ✔ It's more intimate than meeting online or in a group.
>
> ✔ You're obligated to make appointments and come prepared, which holds you accountable.
>
> ✔ You get concrete recommendations within the meeting time frame.

As with other support methods, one-on-one counseling can have pitfalls, such as the following:

- ✔ Failing to follow up will not get you the desired results. You won't get all the answers to your questions and concerns at one visit. Progress is best tracked when working with someone over a period of time.

- ✔ It may take longer to get follow-up appointments (depending on how busy the provider is).

- ✔ You may be uncomfortable revealing important pieces of information when face to face.

Tackling Behavior Change Head On

Although behavior change is essential, it can be challenging. Many behaviors become *habits* (recurrent patterns of behavior acquired through frequent repetition). When you do things on autopilot, like brushing your teeth, tying your shoes, and eating breakfast in the morning, these are habits. The science of habits shows that these repeated behaviors forge strong neural pathways in our brains that can be difficult to change. If you need to break a habit because it's not good for you, such as smoking, excessive drinking, or overeating, it's possible — it just takes time and patience to establish a new neural pathway.

You didn't gain weight overnight. You aren't going to lose it overnight either. It takes time and patience to allow changes to happen in your life.

Here are some of the challenges of behavior change, which may explain why change may be hard in your own life:

- ✔ **Fear of the unknown:** Stepping outside your comfort zone and delving into new behavioral territory is difficult. What's out there waiting for you? It could be great things!

- ✔ **Fear of lack of control:** Letting go of control is hard because it allows for the unknown to happen, but that can be a positive thing in the long run.

- ✔ **Fear of failure:** What happens if you don't succeed at your behavior change right away? You get back on the horse again and take it one day at a time. Before you know it, you'll find success!

In Susan Jeffers's book, *Feel the Fear and Do It Anyway,* she enlightens readers on using fear as motivator to drive you forward versus halting you in your tracks. Fear can be debilitating, but by recognizing it, feeling it, and pushing through it, you'll get to the other side of it, which is a new you full of change and possibility.

Change is a constant, inevitable part of life, yet many people resist it. There's no doubt that you have to be ready to change. If you aren't ready and you're resistant to change, it's not the right time to make the change. Here are some signs that you may be resistant to change:

✔ You're forgetful.

✔ You complain a lot.

✔ You're always procrastinating.

✔ You're disorganized.

✔ You make excuses for yourself.

✔ You sabotage yourself by missing scheduled therapy sessions or not doing your "homework" between sessions.

On the other hand, here are some indicators that you're full steam ahead and ready to make changes:

✔ You're optimistic.

✔ You're determined.

✔ You have a strong support system in place.

✔ You have plans in place for avoiding setbacks.

✔ You're willing to ask for help.

✔ You've set realistic, doable goals.

There so many ways to tackle changing behaviors. Keep in mind that simple, small changes lead to big results down the road. Change is a process that evolves over time. Over time, small changes add up!

Staying on track with behavior change is the key to success. Falling back into old familiar ways of eating with foods that aren't as healthy or lifestyle habits like sitting on the couch and watching TV as soon as you get home from work can be easy. However, with a system in place to set new habits, you won't *relapse* (go back to old habits).

Here are some things you can do to establish new habits, as well as prevent relapses:

✔ Keep a daily food and activity log. Include gold stars for progress!

✔ Call a friend or family member for support.

✔ Don't let minor setbacks get you down. Think positively and forge ahead.

✔ Define a realistic goal. For example, "I'm going to take a brisk walk today." (Start with a short distance and then increase that over time.)

✔ Plan for progress. Make a grocery list or plan to try a new recipe.

✔ Reward yourself with non-food rewards, such as a massage, facial, or new item of clothing.

Cognitive behavioral therapy to the rescue

You may find that your behaviors are so ingrained that it takes a little more assistance to help create new neural pathways or ways of thinking and acting. *Cognitive behavioral therapy* (CBT) is a type of treatment that looks at the relationship between thoughts, feelings, and behaviors. CBT allows you to work with a professional who is focused on the process of problem solving with goal-setting tools and strategies.

In CBT, goals are

✔ **Specific:** You define your goal in detail. For example, "I am not going to sit on the couch and watch TV at night; I am going to do an activity after work."

✔ **Measurable:** You set the goal and are able to assess your progress. For example, "I am going to be active at least three times a week."

✔ **Achievable in a realistic time frame:** You start by setting the goal for one week and then evaluate at the end of that week.

Another example entails a goal of not eating empty-calorie foods at night. CBT enables you to establish a plan to change what you do when you walk in the door from work and helps you create a list of nutrient-dense foods (instead of empty-calorie foods) to keep in the house. Again, it's about equipping you with realistic, simple ways to attain your goals — and change detrimental, self-sabotaging thinking patterns and behaviors.

According to the *Journal of Affective Disorders,* the majority of online interventions are based on CBT because it has been found to be the most beneficial type of therapy (comprising learning-specific skills and techniques). At the heart of CBT is identifying your *core beliefs* (hidden inner thoughts about yourself) that may be stopping you from making healthy lifestyle changes. Core beliefs are complex — you have to look at the emotions that feed the belief. Here are some examples:

✔ Maybe you feel fear when you eat in public. If so, ask yourself what's driving this fear. Do you not want people seeing what or how much you're eating because you think you're overweight?

✔ Maybe you're angry if there's nothing "healthy" on the menu when you dine out. What's driving this anger? Is it because you feel like you can't make menu substitutions or eat less of a high-calorie food?

✔ Maybe you feel guilty if you eat a piece of chocolate cake because it's not allowed on your weight loss plan. Is this bad feeling about yourself coming from the fact that you feel like you may not be able to get back on track after eating this cake?

Think about it, how do your emotions define who you are — in your mind? Emotions are powerful windows to what you think and say about yourself.

Do your homework

CBT is all about you, and the work you do at home is important! Psychologists who specialize in CBT recommend a process called *self-monitoring*. It allows you to see what's working and not working for you.

Looking at your behavior every day allows you to

✔ Anticipate, prevent, and react to potential lifestyle problems every day

✔ Track the relationship between eating and exercise patterns and weight

✔ Gain immediate accountability

✔ Get help with weight loss and maintenance

You can monitor yourself by jotting down your feelings in a notebook, on a smartphone, or on your computer.

Can you self-monitor right now? Think about what you're eating or drinking, and how you feel about your choices. The more awareness you create around your behaviors, the more apt you'll be to make changes and stick with them.

Being patient: Old habits die hard

It takes time to create new habits. Some research says to give it at least a month, if not more. Don't lose hope — keep plugging away. By slowly making a change a day or even once a week, you'll see that you're reaching small milestones pretty quickly!

In her book *Eat, Drink, and Be Mindful*, Dr. Susan Albers advises readers to make small eating changes by mindfully adapting with an exercise that illustrates how little changes can lead to healthier choices down the road. To work your way gradually toward healthier, fewer highly processed foods in a step-by-step manner, Albers advises to gradually and mindfully make eating changes to adapt slowly over time.

For example, if you like salty chips, check out how much sodium is in your current chip choice. Find one with less sodium. After you get used to that one, try switching to one with even less sodium. As you slowly decrease the salt, your body and tastes will adapt and you'll hardly notice it. Eventually, you'll enjoy the taste of the less salty ones better!

Here are the steps to carving out a new habit:

1. **Decide on a habit you want to change.**

   For example, maybe you want to drink an 8-ounce glass of water when you wake up in the morning to hydrate after your overnight slumber. To help reinforce this behavior change, keep a pitcher of water on the nightstand by your bed.

2. **Repeat the new behavior over and over again.**

   Try for at least three to four weeks.

When the new pathway in your brain is set down and it becomes a habit, it will become second nature.

Old habit pathways in your brain never go away. That's why old habits die hard! You always have to be vigilant to avoid the triggers of old habits (like eating ice cream in front of the TV at night or munching on chips while working on your computer).

What is your plan if you fall off track? Think about the Olympic figure skater who falls during a performance or the toddler learning how to walk. What do they have in common? They get back up again and forge ahead. Life is a series of stops and starts, ups and downs. It's a matter of getting back up and not letting the downs keep you there.

Part III
Total Body Diet Recipes

Five Simple Ways to Liven Up Your Kitchen

- **Invite family and friends over to cook.** You may be in a cooking rut or not be inspired to cook. Let friends and family come to the rescue by having them over. Cooking will be a fun, social activity where everyone can participate in making a new recipe or a family favorite with a new and different twist. Plus, eating in good company is always more fun!

- **Cook from creativity without recipes.** Allow yourself to cook with reckless abandon. Use what you have in your pantry and fridge to create a tasty culinary masterpiece that you can call your own. This takes the pressure off not having the right ingredients and allows you to toss the vegetables you have into a stir-fry or chili. Go meatless by using the beans and nuts in your cabinet or rustle up a broth with various herbs and spices on hand.

- **Buy new kitchen gadgets.** It's always fun to get something novel to use in the kitchen like a microplane, a peeler, or even a special knife. You feel empowered when you have tools in the kitchen that can make meal prep easier and more fun. Even if you get a new-fangled meat thermometer or broil pan, it feels like the meat cooks better — and it seems to taste better, too!

- **Refresh your refrigerator.** Ignorance is bliss when it comes to what's in the recesses of your fridge. However, when you clear out the clutter and toss dated cartons, cans, and bottles, and refresh with new dressings, yogurt, produce, and condiments, you feel better opening the fridge and creating a new eating experience. A clean fridge inspires you to eat well, too.

- **Create cooking ambience with inspiring music.** Next time you're in your kitchen and getting ready to make a meal (or thinking about it), turn on the tunes. Whether you like alternative rock, pop, or classical, let the music move you.

Discover herbs and spices for total body health in an article at www.dummies.com/extras/totalbodydiet.

In this part . . .

✔ Whip up delicious and nutritious meals for breakfast, lunch, and dinner.

✔ Make room in your diet for healthy snacks and desserts.

✔ Understand the benefits of herbs and spices to add flavor and cut the salt, sugar, and excess calories in your meals and snacks.

✔ Get the basics on creating healthful food in your kitchen in minutes.

Chapter 9

Breakfasts

In This Chapter

▶ Revealing why breakfast is important for total body wellness

▶ Combining nutrient-dense foods into your first meal of the day

▶ Crafting simple morning meals to fuel your day

*B*reakfast is literally "breaking the fast" that you go through over night. Ideally, you break the fast with nutrient-dense foods to fuel your mind and body at the start of your day. While you sleep, your body is using the left over calories from the day before to repair and restore it for the next day's activities. So, eating a good breakfast of whole grains, lean proteins, fruits and/or vegetables, lowfat or fat-free dairy products, and healthy fats will ensure that you have enough energy for the day ahead.

Why eat breakfast? Many studies have been done on the benefits of breakfast in adults and children. The research points out that breakfast eaters (who eat nutrient-rich foods not foods with too much added sugar) are better able to

✔ Manage body weight better than non-breakfast eaters

✔ Make healthy food choices throughout the day

✔ Concentrate and perform better in the classroom and at work

✔ Maintain their energy and stamina for daily physical activities (plus, they show improved eye-hand coordination)

Breakfast eaters have been shown to keep weight off. A large database research project called The National Weight Control Registry, which consists of people who have lost at least 30 pounds and kept it off for at least five years, shows that the vast majority of successful participants eat breakfast daily. That's a big case for starting your day with a healthy breakfast!

In this chapter, I fill you in on what constitutes a total body breakfast with recipes that'll get your day off on the right foot!

Getting into the habit of eating a good, balanced breakfast starts with simple ways to make breakfast. Whether you're eating breakfast at home or away, your goal is to balance your first meal of the day. Here are some examples of what foods can fit into your breakfast regimen:

- **Good-quality, lean proteins:** Chicken or turkey sausage (low-sodium varieties, if available), whole eggs or egg substitutes, raw or unsalted nuts, nut butters, seeds, beans and bean spreads like hummus, and soy-based meat alternatives, such as soy sausage or crumbles

- **Whole grains:** Oats, whole-wheat bread, brown rice, whole-grain wraps, and quinoa

- **Colorful vegetables:** Bell peppers, spinach, onions, tomatoes, broccoli, asparagus, and carrots

- **Sweet fruits:** Apples, berries, cranberries, dates, figs, grapefruit, mango, melon, oranges, peaches, pears, and plums

- **Lowfat and fat-free dairy products:** Cheeses like Swiss, provolone, or part-skim mozzarella; milk; and plain, unsweetened yogurt

- **Healthy fats:** Avocado, extra-virgin olive oil, nuts, and seeds

Cereals, Muffins, and Breads

Who doesn't love a muffin bursting with blueberries, freshly baked banana nut bread, or a bowl of hot oatmeal for breakfast? Although these are common breakfast foods in the United States, the trick with the Total Body Diet is to choose healthier options among these foods. You think you're doing your body good by eating the fruit-filled muffin, bread, or oatmeal — well, think again. These foods aren't always the healthy option. Check out the portion size and the ingredients to find their nutritional value.

For example, according to the National Heart, Lung, and Blood Institute's Portion Distortion Quiz, a store-bought 5-ounce blueberry muffin contains about 500 calories. That's 310 calories more than they were 20 years ago! To burn off that additional 310 calories, you'd have to vacuum your house for 1 hour and 30 minutes (and nobody's house is *that* dirty!). To see more examples in this quiz, go to www.choosemyplate.gov/supertracker-tools/portion-distortion.html.

Baking at home can help save calories and allow you to throw healthy ingredients — such as nuts and seeds, whole-grain flour, fresh fruit, and even vegetables — into the mix. Even if you aren't a baker, there are simple ways to save calories and boost the nutrition in these breakfast faves — so you can still enjoy them, but not break the calorie bank doing it!

Here are some better-for-you breakfast baking and flavoring tips:

- ✔ Incorporate whole-wheat flour instead of white, all-purpose flour to boost the fiber and nutrients in batters.

- ✔ Instead of oil and butter, use fruit sauces like apple or mango sauce (you can buy them in squeezable tubes or in bottles in the baking aisle of the grocery store) to make quick breads and muffins. It's an equal exchange (¼ cup oil = ¼ cup fruit sauce). You can even swirl fruit puree into hot oatmeal to sweeten it.

- ✔ Use pure extracts like vanilla, almond, orange, mint, and anise to add delicious flavor without added sugar and extra calories. Add ½ teaspoon to cooked oats, Cream of Wheat, farina, or muffin and quick bread batters.

- ✔ Ground flaxseed or sprinkle chia or hemp seeds into batters to add healthy fat and fiber. Also, toss ¼ cup of raw, unsalted pistachios, walnuts, pecans, or almonds into muffins or quick breads.

- ✔ For portion control, bake with mini muffin tins and mini loaf pans. Use smaller cereal bowls, too.

- ✔ Make sweet and savory quick breads with herbs and spices. Add cinnamon, nutmeg, smoked paprika, and fresh or dried herbs like rosemary and thyme to breads.

- ✔ Whip up plain, old-fashioned oats and flavor it yourself. Use a teaspoon drizzle of honey or agave nectar plus ½ teaspoon cinnamon in 1 cup cooked oats instead of presweetened, flavored oatmeal packets.

Hot Oats with Raspberry Maple Compote

Prep time: 5 min • **Cook time:** 15 min • **Yield:** 1 serving

Ingredients	Directions
½ cup fresh raspberries, rinsed and patted dry 1 tablespoon real maple syrup	**1** In a small saucepan over medium heat, add the raspberries and syrup. Bring to a simmer and mash the berries a bit to make a compote. Remove from the heat.
½ cup plain whole oats 1 cup lowfat milk 1 tablespoon flaked coconut, unsweetened	**2** In a small pot over high heat, place the oats and milk. Bring to a boil; then reduce the heat and simmer while stirring. Remove from the heat when the oats are cooked and thick (refer to package for cooking time).
	3 Transfer the cooked oats into a small bowl, top with the raspberry compote, and sprinkle with coconut flakes. Stir and enjoy while hot.

Per serving: Calories 396 (From Fat 98); Fat 11g (Saturated 7g); Cholesterol 12mg; Sodium 115mg; Carbohydrate 62g (Dietary Fiber 9g); Protein 15g.

Pumpkin Pie Mini Muffins

Prep time: 15 min • **Cook time:** 20 min • **Yield:** 8 servings

Ingredients	Directions
1½ cups white whole-wheat flour	*1* Preheat the oven to 350 degrees. Place paper mini muffin liners into a muffin pan and set aside.
1 teaspoon baking powder	
½ teaspoon baking soda	*2* Sift the flour, baking powder, and baking soda, in a medium bowl. Add the cinnamon, nutmeg, ginger, all-spice, and salt.
1 teaspoon ground cinnamon	
1 teaspoon ground nutmeg	
1 teaspoon ground ginger	*3* In a separate bowl, place the eggs, fruit syrup, pumpkin, milk, butter, and orange zest; beat well. Gently fold in the flour mixture until just blended. With a small spoon, pour the batter into each muffin compartment until three-fourths of the way full.
1 teaspoon all-spice	
½ teaspoon salt	
2 eggs	
¼ cup mango puree, all-fruit, no sugar added	*4* Bake for 20 minutes, or until a toothpick poked into the center of a muffin comes out clean. Let cool on the stovetop for a few minutes. Transfer to a wire cooling rack to cool completely. Enjoy with a dollop of jam or nut butter with a cup of hot tea.
One 15-ounce can pumpkin, unsweetened	
1⅔ cups lowfat milk	
¼ cup unsalted butter, melted and cooled	
1 tablespoon freshly grated orange zest	

Per serving: Calories 189 (From Fat 61); Fat 7g (Saturated 4g); Cholesterol 17mg; Sodium 433mg; Carbohydrate 29g (Dietary Fiber 5g); Protein 6g.

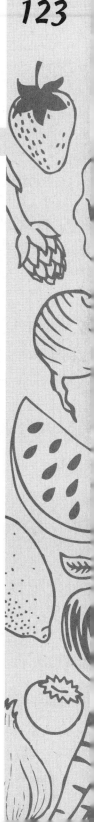

Cinnamon Nut Butter English Muffins

Prep time: 5 min • **Yield:** 1 serving

Ingredients	Directions
1 whole-wheat English muffin	*1* Split the English muffin in half. Put each piece in the toaster until lightly browned.
1 tablespoon natural almond or peanut butter	
1 teaspoon cinnamon	*2* Spread each piece with peanut butter and sprinkle with cinnamon. Enjoy!

Per serving: Calories 235 (From Fat 98); Fat 11g (Saturated 1g); Cholesterol 0mg; Sodium 313mg; Carbohydrate 30g (Dietary Fiber 5g); Protein 8g.

Tip: Use whole-wheat English muffins because they contain more fiber. Look for at least 3g of fiber per muffin. It'll fill you up longer for sustained energy throughout the morning. Feel free to add thinly sliced apples or pears on top for a touch of sweetness and flavor.

Fruit and Vegetable Dishes

Breakfast wouldn't be complete without fruits or vegetables. It may not always be feasible to have both, but adding color, crunch, and vital nutrients in the morning will offer a great jumpstart to your day. If you want to reach the Dietary Guidelines for Americans recommendation of 2½ cups of vegetables and 2 cups of fruits per day, breakfast can be a great step toward that goal.

Think outside the box when it comes to adding produce to breakfast. You can add spinach, tomatoes, and mushrooms to an omelet, or add kale, carrots, and berries into a blender and make a smoothie. Spread a tablespoon of avocado on a slice of whole-grain toast with tomato for a great nutrition boost for the day!

Why fruits and vegetables for breakfast? They offer the following valuable vitamins and minerals:

- **Vitamin C:** Found in citrus fruits and vegetables, vitamin C helps with wound healing.

- **Vitamin A:** Found in leafy greens, as well as carrots, apricots, and sweet potatoes, vitamin A is good for eye health.

- **Beta-carotene:** Found in orange and red fruits and vegetables, beta-carotene may help to reduce the risk of certain cancers and other disease in the body.

- **Vitamin K:** Found in dark leafy greens, avocados, and kiwi, vitamin K helps with wound healing to keep blood clotting normal. Plus, it helps keep your bones healthy.

- **Iron:** Found in leafy greens like spinach and Swiss chard, as well as dried fruits like raisins and apricots, iron gives you energy because it helps provide oxygen to red blood cells. It also helps with focus and memory, and it keeps your immune system functioning well.

- **Folate:** Found in dark leafy greens like spinach, broccoli, and turnip greens, as well as asparagus, oranges, mangoes, and cantaloupe, folate helps with cell growth and metabolism, as well as healthy reproduction. It helps form the central nervous system in developing babies.

Drinking 100 percent juice packed with fruits and vegetables will provide you a lot of nutritional value in the morning, but eating the whole fruits and vegetables will be more satisfying and may even save calories in the long run. Research has shown that *eating* fruits and vegetables (as opposed to drinking them in the form of juice) may keep blood sugar more stable and fend off type-2 diabetes.

Artichoke, Basil, and Yogurt Toast

Prep time: 10 min • **Cook time:** 5 min • **Yield:** 6 servings

Ingredients	Directions
2 cups artichoke hearts, marinated	*1* Drain the artichokes in a colander to remove the excess liquid (but don't rinse to preserve some of the oil and seasonings). In a blender or food processor, add the artichokes, basil, and yogurt. Pulse until combined and the artichokes are still chunky. For some spice, add Sriracha, if desired.
3 fresh basil leaves, washed and patted dry	
½ cup nonfat plain Greek yogurt	
1 teaspoon Sriracha sauce (optional)	*2* Place the artichoke mixture into an 8-inch square broiler-safe baking dish or oval ramekin and top with cheddar cheese. Place in the oven on broil (high heat) for 5 minutes. Check and remove when cheese is melted and golden brown.
2 ounces cheddar cheese, shredded	
6 slices whole-grain bread, toasted	*3* Smear the mixture onto the toast. Enjoy!

Per serving: Calories 273 (From Fat 169); Fat 19g (Saturated 4g); Cholesterol 11mg; Sodium 333mg; Carbohydrate 17g (Dietary Fiber 3g); Protein 9g.

Tip: You can store this mixture in the refrigerator for up to five days.

White Nectarine, Blueberry, and Melon Cottage Cheese Bowl

Prep time: 10 min • **Yield:** 3 servings

Ingredients	Directions
2 large white nectarines, washed, pitted, and diced	*1* In a medium bowl, place the nectarines, berries, and cantaloupe and gently stir to combine.
1 cup blueberries, washed and dried	
1 cup cubed cantaloupe or honeydew melon	*2* Divide the mixture evenly among 3 bowls, and dollop with cottage cheese.
1½ cups lowfat cottage cheese	
1 teaspoon cinnamon	*3* Sprinkle with cinnamon and a drizzle of honey.
1 teaspoon honey	

Per serving: Calories 180 (From Fat 16); Fat 2g (Saturated 1g); Cholesterol 5mg; Sodium 468mg; Carbohydrate 27g (Dietary Fiber 3g); Protein 16g.

Tip: Enjoy with a slice of whole-grain toast with nut butter. You can store the fruit mixture in the refrigerator for up to three days.

Roasted Chile Pepper Ratatouille

Prep time: 25 min • **Cook time:** 20 min • **Yield:** 6 servings

Ingredients	*Directions*
2 medium poblano peppers, seeds and pith removed diced	**1** Wash and dry the produce. Roast the peppers (see the nearby sidebar).
1 tablespoon extra-virgin cold-pressed olive oil	**2** Add the olive oil to a medium saucepan over medium heat; toss in the shallots and cook until translucent, about 5 minutes.
2 small shallots, minced	
4 Roma tomatoes, diced	
2 small zucchini, diced	**3** Add the roasted peppers, tomatoes, zucchini, squash, eggplant, and salt. Stir together until well combined. Cover and let cook for 10 minutes. The vegetables will steam in their own juices. Stir and allow to cook until all vegetable are tender, but not too mushy, for 10 minutes more.
2 small, yellow squash, diced	
1 small eggplant, coarsely diced	
½ teaspoon salt	
Kefir cheese or plain lowfat Greek yogurt (optional)	**4** Top each serving with a small spoonful of kefir cheese or yogurt, if desired.

Per serving: *Calories 93 (From Fat 46); Fat 5g (Saturated 1g); Cholesterol 0mg; Sodium 203mg; Carbohydrate 11g (Dietary Fiber 5g); Protein 3g.*

Tip: Serve on hearty whole-grain crusty bread or add it to scrambled eggs or tofu for a savory breakfast.

How to roast peppers

To roast peppers, follow these simple steps:

1. **Cut the top off each pepper and remove the seeds and white membrane. For more heat, leave the membrane intact, and just remove the seeds.**

2. **Place the seedless peppers over an open flame on the stovetop or grill or under a broiler. Keep an eye on it and rotate as the flesh chars to a brownish black color.**

   Once the whole pepper is charred, remove from the heat.

3. **Immediately place the pepper in a paper bag to sweat. The skin will soften and the burnt layer will separate a bit. Allow to sweat for 5 minutes.**

4. **Remove from the bag and, using a paring knife, remove the charred flesh by rubbing the knife gently over the surface.**

Nut, Egg, and Meat Dishes

Protein-rich foods go a long way toward fueling your body for the day ahead. Research shows that adding protein to breakfast can satisfy your appetite longer, which may help you eat less at lunch and dinner, too.

One of the ways to get good protein, as well as fiber and heart-healthy fats, in the morning is with nuts. Tossing nuts into your breakfast mix offers many nutritional benefits. In Mediterranean cultures, nuts are a powerful player in the daily diet. Many research studies have been devoted to the components of the Mediterranean diet. This way of eating and living incorporates nuts, seeds, fruits, vegetables, whole grains, bean, legumes, and seafood. It may help to promote healthy aging and longevity, heart health, diabetes prevention, and weight control. It may also fend off weight gain around the waistline, which leads to high blood pressure and high cholesterol. Finally, the Mediterranean lifestyle may help reduce the risk of depression, too, because meals are eaten in group settings creating a sense of community.

Eggs are a great source of protein. Crack open an egg and you get a wealth of nutrients from the protein-packed white part to the fatty bright yellow-orange egg yolk, which contains a host of fat-soluble carotenoids, two main ones are lutein and zeaxanthin, which deposit in the retinas of your eyes and have been shown to help keep your eyes young by fending off age-related macular degeneration (AMD).

Choose your breakfast meats wisely. It's easy to get sidetracked with bacon, sausage, and even steak for breakfast. Choose leaner cuts of red meat and pork for breakfast and go meatless more often than not. What are leaner types of breakfast meats? Try Canadian bacon instead of traditional bacon, and chicken or turkey sausage instead of pork sausage.

If you don't eat meat, you can use soy-based meat alternatives like soy sausage and crumbles. They offer a meatlike taste and texture. The pre-seasoned ones may contain too much sodium, so check the labels. Another vegetarian/vegan option is tofu — made from soybeans, it's a complete protein source with low levels of saturated fat and sodium and no cholesterol. Go for the extra-firm type of tofu for breakfast scrambles and bakes.

Kale and Cheddar Omelet

Prep time: 10 min • **Cook time:** 5 min • **Yield:** 1 serving

Ingredients	Directions
1 tablespoon extra-virgin olive oil 2 large garlic cloves, diced 2 cups kale, washed and chopped 2 large eggs, cracked and whisked ¼ cup extra-sharp cheddar, grated A dash of salt and black pepper, to taste Tomato slices (optional) Dijon mustard (optional)	**1** On the stovetop, over medium-low heat, drizzle the oil in a nonstick skillet. Add the garlic and sauté for 1 minute. Add the kale and continue to sauté. Mix and cover to steam the kale a bit. Remove the kale from the skillet and set aside. **2** Pour the eggs into the same skillet and allow their liquid to spread over the entire round surface. Allow to cook until the outer edges become cooked and rise a bit. Add the kale and cheddar (reserve 1 tablespoon for topping). With a spatula, loosen the edges of the cooking eggs by carefully getting under the edges all around. Slowly flip one side over the other half to create an omelet. The bottom should be slightly browned. **3** Top with the reserved tablespoon of cheese, remove from the heat, and cover. Allow the cheese to melt and the eggs to cook for another 30 seconds in the covered skillet. **4** Remove carefully from the skillet with a spatula. Plate your omelet and garnish with sliced tomato and serve with a dollop of Dijon mustard, if desired.

Per serving: Calories 457 (From Fat 308); Fat 34g (Saturated 11g); Cholesterol 453mg; Sodium 529mg; Carbohydrate 17g (Dietary Fiber 3g); Protein 24g.

Thyme Roasted Potato Frittata

Prep time: 25 min • **Cook time:** 35 min • **Yield:** 8 servings

Ingredients	Directions
2 cups diced Yukon Gold potatoes	*1* Preheat the oven to 400 degree.
1 large garlic clove, diced	*2* Toss the potatoes with the garlic, shallots, olive oil, and salt and pepper. Place in an oven-safe baking dish. Roast for 25 minutes and check. If the potatoes are still hard in the center, put them back in the oven for another 15 minutes. Check again; when the flesh is soft and the potatoes are golden brown, remove them from the oven and set aside to cool for a few minutes.
1 small shallot, sliced	
1 tablespoon extra-virgin olive oil	
A pinch of salt and pepper	
1½ teaspoons butter	
5 large eggs, cracked and whisked until frothy and slightly thickened	*3* In a nonstick skillet over medium-low heat, add the butter and allow it to melt. Add the roasted potatoes to sauté for a few minutes. Pour in the eggs and allow them to cover the whole round of the skillet. Sprinkle the thyme, salt, and pepper over the mixture and allow it to set. Turn the heat to low and cover. The eggs will rise a bit as they cook. With a spatula, loosen the sides of the eggs from the skillet and work it toward the middle to stop it from sticking (and to check the browning of the bottom). Sprinkle on the cheese and cover again. Allow the center to solidify and quickly remove from the heat. Using a spatula, gently outline the sides and work toward the middle. It should loosen easily; lay it on a serving plate.
1 to 2 sprigs of thyme, washed and leaves removed	
Salt and pepper, to taste	
¼ cup parmesan cheese shavings	
2 teaspoons Dijon mustard (optional)	
	4 Serve immediately while warm. Dip each forkful in a dollop of Dijon mustard, if desired.

Per serving: Calories 108 (From Fat 59); Fat 7g (Saturated 2g); Cholesterol 137mg; Sodium 201mg; Carbohydrate 7g (Dietary Fiber 1g); Protein 6g.

Sweet and Spicy Almonds

Prep time: 15 min • **Cook time:** 10 min • **Yield:** 9 servings

Ingredients	Directions
1½ cups raw almonds	*1* In a medium nonstick sauté pan, toss the almonds over medium heat. Heat until fragrant and beginning to brown (about 5 to 10 minutes). Shake the pan to toss the nuts a bit while heating. Remove from the heat.
2 teaspoons honey	
1 teaspoon ground cinnamon	
1 teaspoon ground nutmeg	
1 teaspoon unsweetened cocoa powder	*2* Drizzle the nuts with honey and mix with a spoon to coat. Sprinkle with cinnamon, nutmeg, cocoa powder, and salt, if desired. Toss together and add the coconut, raisins, and cranberries.
½ teaspoon salt (optional)	
2 teaspoons unsweetened flaked coconut	
1 tablespoon raisins	*3* Place in a bowl or store in a tin or air-tight plastic container in a dry, cool place. Spoon a tablespoon over oatmeal or into your favorite whole-grain cereal.
1 tablespoon dried cranberries	

Per serving: Calories 153 (From Fat 112); Fat 12g (Saturated 1g); Cholesterol 0mg; Sodium 1mg; Carbohydrate 8g (Dietary Fiber 3g); Protein 5g.

Yogurt and Cheese Dishes

Dairy products like yogurt and cheese are big breakfast foods. They're rich in protein and calcium, but you have to watch the saturated fats in full-fat yogurts and cheeses. Choose lowfat or fat-free options, whenever possible. (If you eat full-fat versions occasionally, just choose smaller portion sizes.)

With the myriad of yogurts on the grocery stores shelves, it's easy to get caught with varieties that have a lot of added sugar in your shopping cart. The solution: Check the Nutrition Facts panel on the containers to make sure there isn't a lot of added sugar listed in the ingredients. The best bet is to buy plain lowfat yogurt and add your own sweet touch with a drizzle of honey, agave nectar, berries, or cut-up fruit.

Even plain, unsweetened yogurt contains sugar. That's because yogurt — and all milk products — naturally contain a milk sugar called lactose. Look at the ingredient list for sugar or some other sweetener such as fructose, honey, or Florida crystals, especially within the first five ingredients. Greek and Icelandic yogurts have more protein because they're strained, which removes excess water.

Also, look for "live, active cultures" on the label to ensure that there are probiotics or friendly bacteria in the yogurt, which add to the microflora of your gut and help keep you healthy.

Make your own Greek yogurt

If you want to make your own Greek yogurt, which is strained to remove the whey protein, here's what you do:

1. Place a fine sieve or colander over an empty bowl with a cheese cloth in it.

2. Spoon the regular, plain yogurt into it and allow it to strain.

3. Place the bowl in the refrigerator for two hours or more to allow the liquid to fully strain out.

Note: One cup of regular yogurt will make ½ cup of Greek-style, thick yogurt. If you plan to strain your own yogurt often, you can purchase a yogurt strainer.

As the yogurt thickens, the whey protein will be left behind (in the bowl). You can save the whey protein (a yellowish liquid with a sour taste) — it contains a lot of nutrients. Put it in the refrigerator and it'll last for a week. You can add it to homemade pizza dough, cook oatmeal or quinoa in it for added protein, or use it as the liquid for baking quick breads.

Cheese is a go-to food for breakfast. Whether on bread, in eggs, or tossed into casseroles, it offers hearty, rich flavor as well as satisfying protein and fat. A little goes a long way, though. A serving is equivalent to 1½ ounces of hard cheese or 2 ounces of processed cheese. Sprinkling on grated cheese, slicing it thinly, or cutting it into small cubes is the way to control the portion, yet still enjoy the richness that cheese imparts.

Here are some ideas on ways to get cheese and yogurt in at breakfast:

- ✔ Grab a cup of plain, lowfat yogurt with fresh berries and ¼ cup of whole-grain cereal.

- ✔ Melt a slice of Swiss cheese on whole-grain bread with a slice of tomato.

- ✔ Mix an ounce of grated part-skim mozzarella cheese into a whisked egg and scramble on the stovetop.

- ✔ Drizzle a teaspoon of honey and sprinkle cinnamon on top of nonfat plain Greek or regular yogurt.

- ✔ Sprinkle 2 ounces of grated part-skim mozzarella cheese on a homemade egg, bell pepper, and tomato breakfast burrito.

Garlic Herb Cheddar and Tomato Melt

Prep time: 5 min • **Cook time:** 5 min • **Yield:** 1 serving

Ingredients	Directions
1½ teaspoons unsalted butter	**1** Place butter in a small sauté pan over medium heat; melt and coat pan. Pile the greens, tomato, and cheese on the bread and place into the pan with the cheese side up.
5 baby green leaves, washed and dried	
1 small plum tomato, washed and sliced thinly	**2** Cover the pan and heat through until the cheese is melted and beginning to brown. (You can also place in a broiler oven; the cheese will bubble and brown nicely!)
1 ounce garlic herb cheddar cheese	
1 slice whole-grain bread	**3** With a spatula, remove from the pan and put on a plate. Enjoy immediately.

Per serving: Calories 245 (From Fat 147); Fat 16g (Saturated 10g); Cholesterol 45mg; Sodium 289mg; Carbohydrate 14g (Dietary Fiber 3g); Protein 11g.

Strawberry, Hemp Seed, and Cinnamon Yogurt Swirl

Prep time: 5 min • **Yield:** 4 servings

Ingredients	Directions
4 cups nonfat plain Greek yogurt	**1** Place the yogurt, strawberries, hemp seeds, and cinnamon in a blender or food processor and pulse until combined.
2 cups strawberries, washed and diced	
2 tablespoon hemp seeds	**2** Spoon into 4 parfait glasses. Drizzle with honey or agave nectar, if desired.
2 teaspoons cinnamon	
1 teaspoon honey or agave nectar (optional)	

Per serving: Calories 186 (From Fat 29); Fat 3g (Saturated 3g); Cholesterol 12mg; Sodium 84mg; Carbohydrate 16g (Dietary Fiber 3g); Protein 24g.

Tip: Store leftover parfaits in the refrigerator, covered with plastic wrap for up to a week.

Grape Juice Glazed Almond Ricotta Cheese Cups

Prep time: 5 min • **Cook time:** 20 min • **Yield:** 8 servings

Ingredients	Directions
1 cup 100 percent grape juice	**1** Preheat the oven to 350 degrees.
1 teaspoon honey	
1 cup slivered raw almonds	**2** In a medium nonstick saucepan over high heat, add the juice and honey. Bring to a boil and then simmer. Stir frequently to thicken. Toss in the almonds and coat thoroughly. Remove from the heat and place on a baking sheet covered with parchment paper. Spread out and bake the glazed nuts in the oven for 10 minutes, until golden brown. Remove from the oven and let cool. Sprinkle with cinnamon. (Store the remainder of the almonds in an air-tight container in the fridge or a cool dark place.)
1 teaspoon cinnamon (for dusting)	
4 cups part-skim ricotta cheese	
	3 Put ½ cup of ricotta cheese into eight individual cups. Spoon the nut mixture over the ricotta cheese cups. Enjoy immediately or place in the refrigerator for up to 3 days.

Per serving: Calories 269 (From Fat 148); Fat 16g (Saturated 7g); Cholesterol 38mg; Sodium 156mg; Carbohydrate 15g (Dietary Fiber 2g); Protein 17g.

Note: Wait to top the ricotta with nuts until you're ready to eat it.

Chapter 10

Lunches

In This Chapter

▶ Jazzing up your midday meals in healthy and tasty ways

▶ Uncovering balance on your plate without boredom

▶ Learning to pack energizing meals to enhance productivity for the day

*E*ver have the feeling of wanting to fall asleep at your desk after a heavy lunch? Or maybe you didn't eat enough — and the few handfuls of popcorn and diet soda you scarfed down at noon just didn't cut it. Eating a balanced lunch is essential to fuel your mind and body well for the work ahead — whether it's at the office, running around with the kids, or studying. Your midday meal sets the tone for the rest of the day.

Want to make healthy lunches that you can bring with you on the go? Incorporate high-fiber carbohydrates, lean protein, and healthy fats. Not only will you feel more satisfied, but you'll have better energy, boosted brain power, and more productivity throughout the day!

Here are some tips to plan and pack healthy lunches:

> ✔ **Make it portable.** Use plastic containers with compartments for sandwiches, wraps, salads, veggies, fruits, and cheese.

> ✔ **Contain the heat.** Bring soups and veggie chili in thermos containers. A good rule of thumb is to fill your thermos with boiling hot water, and then empty it and fill it with piping hot food.

✔ **Keep cold foods cold with ice packs and refrigerate sandwiches that include cold cuts; fruits; yogurt; cheese; salads; dairy or mayo-based egg, chicken, or tuna salads; and beverages.** If you can, store perishable items in the refrigerator. Perishable foods should not be kept at room temperature more than two hours including prep time.

✔ **Plan your lunches, just like any other meal.** If you know that you're going out to lunch, think about what you're going to order and where you're going beforehand.

Soup's On!

You can't go wrong with soup — hot or cold. Not only is soup a hydrating liquid, but it's a nutrient-dense meal with a blend of healthy ingredients, which may include vegetables, fruits, beans, peas, protein from poultry, seafood, lean meat, or tofu, as well as lowfat or fat-free dairy products. Plus, many soups are packed with herbs and spices, which provide an additional nutrition boost without added sodium or calories. It's not only an easy meal, but you can make soup ahead of time in large batches to enjoy for days and freeze for weeks ahead.

From Italian minestrone soup to Moroccan lentil soup to Thai tom yum soup, every culture has soup on the menu because it nourishes the mind and body with vital nutrients — and it's simple to make. Just toss ingredients in a pot and allow it to cook, or puree ingredients together for soups that be eaten cold. Chunky or smooth, soup allows you to craft a unique flavor profile to suit your taste buds.

Of course, some soups are better for you than others. Here are some of the healthier soups:

✔ **Broth-based soups:** These soups usually contain more water and less fat and calories. (Watch the sodium, though!) Some examples of broth-based soups include miso soup and chicken noodle soup.

✔ **Vegetable- and fruit-based soups:** These soups contain more nutrients and fewer calories. Some examples include beet soup, gazpacho, and minestrone.

✔ **Bean-based soups:** These soups contain more fiber and protein, and have a moderate calorie count. Some examples include black bean soup and lentil soup.

Here are some examples of less-healthy soups to watch out for:

✔ **Cream-based soups:** These soups are usually made from cream, which contains more saturated fat and calories. Some examples of cream-based soups include cream of corn soup, cream of mushroom soup, and creamy tomato soup.

✔ **Meat-based soups:** These soups have more calories and are higher in saturated fat and sodium. Some examples of meat-based soups include sausage gumbo and bacon soup.

✔ **Cheesy soups:** These soups are higher in saturated fat, calories, and sodium. Some examples of cheesy soups include French onion soup.

The basis of a good soup is broth (also known as stock). You can purchase premade broth at any grocery store, but making it yourself is more nutritious because you use fresh ingredients and control how much salt is added. When buying broth, look for *low-sodium* or *no-salt added* on the label — you can always add a pinch or two of salt for taste if you want.

Spicy Tomato Basil Ricotta Soup

Prep Time: 5 min • **Cook Time:** 15–20 min • **Yield:** 2 servings

Ingredients	Directions
8 whole ripe Roma tomatoes, stem removed	**1** In a blender, place the tomatoes and broth. Puree the ingredients and transfer the liquid to a pot. Heat over medium heat for 10 minutes.
½ cup low-sodium vegetable or chicken broth	
2 tablespoons part-skim ricotta cheese	**2** Divide soup evenly between 2 bowls and dollop each with 1 tablespoon ricotta cheese and ½ teaspoon Sriracha and stir. Sprinkle with basil. Serve immediately with bread, if desired.
1 teaspoon Sriracha (hot chili sauce)	
6 fresh basil leaves, sliced into thin strips, or 1 tablespoon dried basil	
2 pieces whole-grain crusty bread (optional)	

Per serving: Calories 74 (From Fat 17); Fat 2g (Saturated 1g); Cholesterol 4mg; Sodium 167mg; Carbohydrate 11g (Dietary Fiber 3g); Protein 5g.

Tip: Sriracha, a spicy chili sauce made from sun-ripened chile peppers, has become a hot (no pun intended) condiment in recent years. A small squirt goes a long way, so use it sparingly at first to tame the heat. If you want a smoky flavor — and less spiciness — you can use a few pinches of Spanish smoked paprika instead.

Curried Broccoli Almond Soup

Prep Time: 5 min • **Cook Time:** 15–20 min • **Yield:** 2 servings

Ingredients	Directions
1 large head broccoli (including florets and most of the stalk), washed and coarsely chopped **½ cup raw almonds** **1 cup lowfat milk** **¼ cup water (optional)** **1 teaspoon curry powder** **Pinch of salt**	*1* In a colander over boiling water, steam broccoli for 5 to 7 minutes (until vibrant green) and remove from heat. (If you prefer, you can also place the broccoli in the microwave, uncovered, for 60 to 90 seconds — no water needed.) Let cool for a minute. *2* Transfer broccoli to a blender. Add almonds, milk, water (for a thinner consistency), curry powder, and salt. Cover and puree for 1 to 2 minutes. Transfer to a small saucepan, bring to a simmer, and heat for 5 minutes. Remove from heat, divide soup evenly between 2 bowls, and serve. Place remaining soup in the freezer for later use.

Per serving: Calories 309 (From Fat 164); Fat 20g (Saturated 2g); Cholesterol 6mg; Sodium 345mg; Carbohydrate 25g (Dietary Fiber 9g); Protein 15g.

Remember: When steaming broccoli be careful not to overcook it because you'll lose vital nutrients, as well as flavor. The broccoli heads should be vibrant green and the stalks firm, not mushy, when done. (When you boil vegetables, nutrients can be lost in the water, so steaming or microwaving is your best bet for retaining nutrients.)

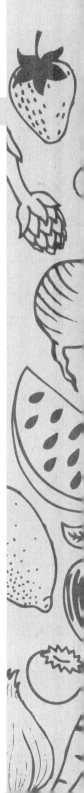

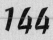

Chicken and Lentil Soup

Prep Time: 5 min • **Cook Time:** 30–40 min • **Yield:** 4 servings

Ingredients

1 tablespoon olive oil

One 4-ounce chicken breast, cut into bite-size pieces

1 medium celery stalk, diced

1 medium carrot, peeled and diced

½ yellow onion, diced

3 garlic cloves, minced

½ teaspoon salt

½ teaspoon ground black pepper

1 quart low-sodium vegetable broth

One 15.5-ounce can diced (no-salted added) tomatoes, undrained

1¼ cup dry lentils, rinsed

1 bay leaf

¼ teaspoon fresh thyme, chopped

1 teaspoon red wine vinegar

2 cups spinach leaves, washed and dried

Salt and pepper (optional)

Directions

1 In a large saucepan, heat oil over medium heat. Add chicken pieces and sauté for 10 minutes or until chicken turns white and golden brown. Add celery, carrot, and onion. Stir occasionally until vegetables begin to soften, about 10 minutes.

2 Stir in garlic and cook until fragrant, about 1 minute. Season with salt and pepper.

3 Add vegetable broth, tomatoes (with juice), lentils, bay leaf, and thyme and stir to combine. Cover and simmer about 15 minutes. Once simmering, reduce heat to low and continue to simmer, covered, about 15 minutes until lentils are soft.

4 Stir in vinegar and spinach until wilted. Season with salt and pepper as needed.

Per serving: Calories 342 (From Fat 58); Fat 6g (Saturated 1g); Cholesterol 18mg; Sodium 427mg; Carbohydrate 48g (Dietary Fiber 20g); Protein 28g.

Sandwich Time

As American as apple pie, the sandwich is a staple at lunchtime — or any time of day, for that matter. The great thing about a sandwich is you can get creative with the type of bread and fillings you use and make it a healthy part of your lunch.

Here are some healthy ways to compile a better-for-you sandwich:

- Start with whole-grain bread or *sandwich thin* (a round, slim, sliced bread that is perfect for holding most any filling) because you'll be adding fiber, iron, folate, and magnesium.

- Power it up with good-quality protein like nut butter, chicken or turkey breast, roast beef, hummus, eggs, seafood, and tofu.

- Fill in with some healthy fats like ripe avocado, olive oil, chopped olives or nuts, or seeds.

- Crunch it up with fruits and vegetables like cucumbers, tomatoes, bell peppers, pickles, broccoli, apples, pears, and plums.

- Spice it up with less fat and calories with mustards, curry powder, Sriracha (spicy chile sauce), smoked paprika, minced garlic, or ginger.

Don't fall into sandwich traps, such as high-fat condiments like mayonnaise or *aioli* (an egg and oil-based dressing); creamy dressings like ranch or Thousand Island; processed meats like salami, pepperoni, pastrami, or corned beef; thick white breads, rolls, and buns; sugar-laden barbecue sauce; and ketchup. All these can add up to excess empty calories from solid fat and added sugars. When in doubt, ask for condiments and dressings on the side, a small sandwich (6-inch instead of a 12-inch sub), and a whole-grain bread.

Apple and Chipotle Cheddar Sandwich

Prep Time: 5 min • **Yield:** 1 serving

Ingredients	Directions
2 slices whole-grain bread	*1* Lay the bread slices out and spread the mustard on both slices.
1 tablespoon chipotle mustard	
¼ medium apple, thinly sliced	*2* Top one slice with apple, cheese, and lettuce. Place the other slice of bread on top to make a sandwich. Cut in half and enjoy!
1 ounce cheddar cheese, thinly sliced	
1 romaine lettuce leaf, washed and dried	

Per serving: Calories 286 (From Fat 110); Fat 12g (Saturated 6g); Cholesterol 30mg; Sodium 565mg; Carbohydrate 30g (Dietary Fiber 5g); Protein 15g.

Tip: You can purchase chipotle-flavored mustard or make your own by simply tossing ½ teaspoon crushed chipotle pepper flakes (or grind them in a spice grinder) into brown mustard. Mix and spread generously on bread, tortillas for wraps, or sandwich thins.

Curried Salmon and Greens Sandwich

Prep Time: 5 min • **Yield:** 1 serving

Ingredients	*Directions*
One 5-ounce can wild salmon, packed in water and drained	*1* In a small bowl, add salmon, scallions, curry powder, mustard, and yogurt. Mix.
1 tablespoon scallions, sliced	
1 teaspoon curry powder	*2* Cut the sandwich thin in half. Pile greens over half of the sandwich thin and dollop with the salmon mixture. Top with the other half. Enjoy!
1 teaspoon Dijon mustard	
1 tablespoon plain lowfat Greek yogurt	
1 sandwich thin	
¼ cup baby greens, washed and dried	

Per serving: Calories 331 (From Fat 108); Fat 12g (Saturated 3g); Cholesterol 63mg; Sodium 363mg; Carbohydrate 22g (Dietary Fiber 4g); Protein 34g.

Note: If you want to use fresh salmon, simply put a salmon filet on a foil-lined cookie sheet or baking dish and place in a preheated oven at 375 degrees. Cook for 5 to 7 minutes and check for doneness by putting a food thermometer in the thickest part of the fish. It's done when the internal temperature is 145 degrees. Remove from the oven and let rest for a few minutes before use.

Mediterranean Reuben Sandwich

Prep Time: 5 min • **Cook Time:** 10 min • **Yield:** 1 serving

Ingredients	Directions
1 teaspoon extra-virgin olive oil	**1** In a sauté pan over medium-low heat, add oil and coat the pan.
2 tablespoons olive tapenade spread	**2** Spread the tapenade on one slice of bread. Add the sauerkraut, cheese, and turkey breast, and cover with the other slice of bread.
2 slices whole-grain bread	
½ cup low-sodium sauerkraut, well drained	
1 slice Swiss cheese	**3** Place the sandwich in the heated sauté pan on the stove and cover. In a minute, check and flip with a heat-proof spatula. Toast both sides and melt the cheese. Serve immediately.
3 ounces low-sodium turkey breast	

Per serving: Calories 412 (From Fat 166); Fat 18g (Saturated 6g); Cholesterol 61mg; Sodium 876mg; Carbohydrate 31g (Dietary Fiber 7g); Protein 31g.

Get Your Midday Salad Fix

There's no better time to eat a salad than at lunchtime. This is an easy way to get the recommended daily dose for adults of 2 to 3 cups of vegetables and 1½ to 2 cups of fruit. The best part is you can get creative with your salads and throw in everything from greens to beans to grains to cheese to chicken. However, be careful — just because it's a salad, doesn't mean it's good for your waistline. Salads with ingredients like bacon, a lot of cheese and nuts, dressing, and croutons can be high in calories and saturated fat.

Here are some ways to create healthy salads that are tasty and won't break your calorie budget:

- **Begin with a base of dark-green leafy vegetables.** They're not only low in calories, but jam-packed with nutrients like iron, calcium, folate, and potassium — all of which bodes well for your total body wellness.

- **Go crazy adding more veggies and fruits.** Try broccoli, tomatoes, carrots, bell peppers, asparagus, berries, mandarin oranges, melon, pineapple, and kiwi.

- **Opt for lean protein.** Try cooked, shredded chicken and turkey breast or pork, baked or grilled seafood, grilled sirloin strips, tofu cubes, or beans.

- **Gently add whole grains.** One-half cup cooked is the equivalent of a 1-ounce serving. Add a serving of quinoa, brown rice, whole-grain pasta, or wheat berries.

- **Factor in healthy fat, but use less by measuring.** For example, a serving of avocado is ½ of a medium one. A serving of nuts and seeds is 1 ounce. And a serving of olive oil is 1 tablespoon.

- **Use cheese sparingly.** It can be high in calories and saturated fat. Your best bet is to grate cheese into your salads like Parmesan, Romano, and part-skim mozzarella. You can always look for lowfat version of Swiss, cottage cheese, ricotta, and cheddar cheese.

If you're making chicken, tuna, salmon, or egg salad, use plain, lowfat Greek yogurt instead of mayonnaise to cut the fat. Plus, yogurt adds protein and calcium. Add diced scallions, Dijon mustard, and herbs like dill or rosemary to the salad, and put the salad on a bed of baby greens.

Spinach, Chicken, and Goat Cheese Spinach Bowl

Prep Time: 10 min • **Cook Time:** 20 min • **Yield:** 2 servings

Ingredients	Directions
½ cup quinoa, rinsed	**1** In a saucepan over high heat, bring quinoa and water to a boil. Add salt and olive oil. Lower the heat and simmer, covered, for about 15 minutes or until water is absorbed. Fluff with a fork and set aside.
1 cup water	
Pinch of salt	
1 tablespoon extra-virgin olive oil	**2** In a large sauté pan over medium heat, add the sunflower seeds and toast for 2 minutes, stirring occasionally.
2 tablespoons unsalted raw sunflower seeds	
2 garlic cloves, minced	**3** Add the garlic to the pan and cook until fragrant, about 1 minute. Add the chicken, quinoa, and spinach to sauté pan and combine. Cook until the spinach is wilted. Then add the lemon juice.
1 cup diced and cooked chicken breast	
1 cup spinach leaves, washed and dried	
3 tablespoons lemon juice	**4** Remove from the heat and toss with the goat cheese and pepper. Divide evenly between 2 bowls and serve.
2 tablespoons goat cheese	
Pinch of ground black pepper	

Per serving: Calories 382 (From Fat 135); Fat 15g (Saturated 3g); Cholesterol 63mg; Sodium 84mg; Carbohydrate 32g (Dietary Fiber 4g); Protein 30g.

Zucchini, Beets, Romaine Hearts, and Feta Salad

Prep Time: 15 min • **Cook Time:** 15 min • **Yield:** 1 serving

Ingredients	Directions
1 small zucchini, sliced	**1** Heat a griddle or grill pan over medium-high heat. Place the sliced zucchini in the pan and brush both sides lightly with the olive oil and sprinkle with salt and pepper. Cook until grill marks appear and the zucchini softens, about 5 minutes on each side. Remove from the grill, let cool, and dice.
1 tablespoon extra-virgin olive oil	
Pinch of salt and black pepper	
2 cups romaine hearts, washed and shredded	**2** In a salad bowl, place the romaine, beets, and zucchini and sprinkle with feta cheese and giardiniera to spice it up, if desired. Serve.
2 small cooked red beets, peeled and diced	
1 tablespoon feta cheese	
1 teaspoon hot giardiniera (optional)	

Per serving: Calories 112 (From Fat 73); Fat 8g (Saturated 2g); Cholesterol 4mg; Sodium 283mg; Carbohydrate 9g (Dietary Fiber 3g); Protein 3g.

Note: No dressing is needed for this salad because the grilled zucchini and giardiniera add oil and flavor. If you want, enjoy the salad with a slice of crusty whole-grain bread or grilled lean meat, such as skirt steak, flank steak, or pork loin.

Tip: Giardiniera is a relish-style condiment consisting of a blend of hot or mild pickled peppers and vegetables (celery, carrots, cauliflower, olives) in oil or vinegar. It's used in sandwiches, soups, chili, salads, omelets, and bruschetta.

Pea, Cucumber, Cipollini Onion, and Mint Salad

Prep Time: 15 min • **Cook Time:** 10 min • **Yield:** 2 servings

Ingredients	Directions
2½ tablespoons extra-virgin olive oil	**1** Place a small sauté pan over medium heat and add ½ tablespoon of the olive oil and the onions. Sauté the onions until golden brown. Set aside.
3 Cipollini onions, sliced	
2 cups sliced mini cucumbers	**2** In a medium bowl, toss together the cucumbers and peas.
1 cup petite peas, thawed (if frozen)	
2 tablespoons balsamic vinegar	**3** In a small bowl, whisk together the remaining olive oil, vinegar, mustard, salt, and pepper. Drizzle the dressing on top of the cucumbers and peas and toss; top with the onions and mint. Top with a few shavings of cheddar cheese. Serve.
1 teaspoon Dijon mustard	
Dash of salt and pepper	
4 fresh mint leaves, coarsely chopped	
A few shavings of sharp cheddar cheese	

Per serving: Calories 259 (From Fat 166); Fat 18g (Saturated 3g); Cholesterol 4mg; Sodium 179mg; Carbohydrate 19g (Dietary Fiber 4g); Protein 6g.

Note: Cipollini onions look like small Vidalia onions.

Chapter 11

Dinners

In This Chapter

▶ Discovering total body diet dinners that are quick and simple to make

▶ Creating evening meals that won't break your calorie bank

▶ Balancing your dinners with healthy ingredients

*T*he last meal of the day may not seem as important as the first, but after a long day, getting the nutrients your body needs to restore and replenish itself is vital. However, because your body slows down in the evening to accommodate your natural sleep cycle, it's important not to overdo it with excess calories after dark.

Here are a few healthy habits to get into for dinnertime:

✔ **Eat earlier in the evening to give your body a chance to digest.** Evenings can be hectic and getting a meal on the table can be stressful, if you haven't planned ahead. Making simple meals ahead of time or knowing what you're going to eat prevents unhealthy eating.

✔ **Balance meals with all the foods groups** — lean protein, fruits and vegetables, whole grains, and/or lowfat dairy products and some healthy fats — for a moderate dinner that fuels your body well for the seven- to nine-hour fast ahead, restorative rest for your mind and body, and rejuvenation for the next day.

✔ **Eat light at night.** The saying, "Eat like a king in the morning, a prince in the afternoon, and a pauper at night" has a lot of truth to it. Try to eat most of your food earlier in the day because you're typically more active during the day, and your metabolism is humming along well — which bodes well for weight management over the long run.

✔ **Eat mindfully in the evening.** Sit down, savor your food, and turn off the outside world. By taking the time with your meal at night, you start the latter part of your day in a restful way. Without distractions, you can fully taste your food, participate in the meal, and connect with your hunger and fullness better. Food is more satisfying when you eat with mindful intention instead of gobbling it down. And when you're satisfied by your meal, you won't feel the need to eat more and more.

Vegetable and Bean Dishes

There's no better time to get your vegetables and beans in than at dinner-time. They make for lighter meals that are packed with fiber, protein, and nutrients. Incorporating more plant foods in your diet is not only beneficial for your total body health (potassium keeps blood pressure in check, fiber helps manage cholesterol, antioxidants are great for cell health), but can also help you manage your waistline because plant foods contain fewer calories and less fat and fill you up longer.

Here are some simple ways to make vegetables and beans a tasty dinner:

✔ Buy vegetables in steamer bags. Just pop them in the microwave and then toss them into whole grains like quinoa, brown rice, or whole wheat pasta.

✔ Defrost frozen vegetables like broccoli and cauliflower florets, diced bell peppers, potatoes, and carrots along with edamame. Then add a can of diced tomatoes and heat together to make vegetable chili.

✔ Toss any type of canned beans (rinse and drain before use) over mixed greens, cherry tomatoes, and mini cucumbers. Top with a drizzle of vin-aigrette for a tasty, hearty salad.

✔ Roast vegetables like zucchini, yellow squash, eggplant, Brussels sprouts, and shallots together and toss with red kidney and white can-nellini beans for a colorful meal that's filling and nutritious.

Making vegetables and beans part of your dinner repertoire is just as easy as relying on meat. Offering your body plant-based meals is a great way to jumpstart your road to total body wellness. The best part is you don't need complex recipes to make healthy, balanced meals. The ones in this section are a great place to start!

Green Tea Quinoa Asian Lettuce Cups

Prep time: 5 min • **Cook time:** 15 min • **Yield:** 4 servings

Ingredients	Directions
1 green tea bag	**1** Place about 1½ cups of water in a small saucepan and bring to a boil. Take it off the heat, add the green tea bag, and let steep for at least 3 to 4 minutes. Remove the tea bag.
1¼ cups, quinoa, rinsed	
1 tablespoon sesame oil	
1 tablespoon low-sodium soy sauce	**2** Add the quinoa to the liquid tea. Bring to a boil. Lower the heat and let simmer for 5 to 10 minutes or until the liquid is absorbed and the quinoa can be fluffed easily with a fork. Remove from heat.
½ lemon or lime, squeezed for juice	
¼ cup cilantro, minced or chopped	**3** In the pot with the quinoa, stir in the oil, soy sauce, lemon or lime juice, cilantro, and carrots. Toss together and divide evenly among the lettuce cups. Eat immediately (no utensils required).
¼ cup carrots, diced	
4 romaine or bibb lettuce leaves, washed and air dried	

Per serving: Calories 233 (From Fat 60); Fat 7g (Saturated 1g); Cholesterol 0mg; Sodium 145mg; Carbohydrate 36g (Dietary Fiber 4g); Protein 8g.

Tip: When making hot tea, begin with purified, filtered water, if possible. To avoid astringent taste, the water should be just at the boiling point (no more than 180 degrees). Steep tea at least 3 minutes to get the maximum antioxidants.

Sweet Potato, Black Bean, and Goat Cheese Tacos

Prep time: 10 min • **Cook time:** 25 min • **Yield:** 6 servings

Ingredients	Directions
2 tablespoons extra-virgin olive oil	**1** In a medium skillet, add the oil and sweet potatoes; sauté for about 10 minutes.
2 cups peeled and diced sweet potatoes	
½ cup finely diced red onion	**2** Add the onions to the skillet and sauté for about 10 more minutes. Add the garlic and cumin, and stir for approximately 1 minute.
2 cloves garlic, minced	
1 teaspoon cumin	
½ teaspoon dried oregano	**3** Add the oregano, beans, and reserved liquid to the skillet and simmer for 10 minutes. (If the mixture gets dry, add 3 tablespoons of water). Combine with the potato and onion mixture and drizzle with lime juice.
One 15-ounce can black beans, drained (reserve 2 tablespoons of liquid from the can)	
Juice of ¼ fresh lime	**4** Fill the tortillas with the sweet potato–black bean mixture. Garnish with goat cheese, cilantro, and avocado.
Six 6-inch corn tortillas	
1 ounce goat cheese	
3 to 4 sprigs fresh cilantro, coarsely chopped	
1 medium avocado, diced	

Per serving: Calories 247 (From Fat 91); Fat 10g (Saturated 2g); Cholesterol 4mg; Sodium 232mg; Carbohydrate 34g (Dietary Fiber 9g); Protein 7g.

Thai Cucumber Brown Rice Bowls

Prep time: 15 min • **Cook time:** 1 hr • **Yield:** 3 servings

Ingredients	Directions
1 cup brown basmati rice	**1** In a medium-size pot over high heat, add the rice and water. Bring to a boil and reduce the heat to a simmer; stir the rice and cover. Simmer for about 45 minutes. Remove from the heat and let stand covered for 5 to 10 minutes more.
2¼ cups water	
6 mini cucumbers, thinly sliced	
2 scallions, sliced	**2** In a large bowl, combine the cucumbers, scallions, and cilantro.
½ cup cilantro leaves, coarsely chopped	
2 tablespoons sesame oil	**3** In a small mixing bowl, add the sesame oil, fish sauce, juice from the two lime halves, agave nectar or honey, and Sriracha sauce. Whisk together until blended.
1 teaspoon Thai fish sauce	
1 large lime, halved	
2 teaspoons agave nectar or honey	**4** Divide the cooked rice evenly among 3 bowls. Top with cucumber salad. Sprinkle with bell pepper bits and sesame seeds (if desired).
1 teaspoon Sriracha sauce	
1 small red bell pepper, chopped	
1 teaspoon sesame seeds (optional)	

Per serving: Calories 355 (From Fat 101); Fat 11g (Saturated 2g); Cholesterol 0mg; Sodium 161mg; Carbohydrate 58g (Dietary Fiber 4g); Protein 6g.

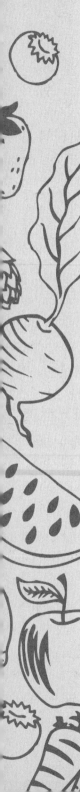

Rosemary Lentils and Tomato Stuffed Peppers

Prep time: 15 min • **Cook time:** 1 hr • **Yield:** 3 servings

Ingredients	Directions
3 large bell peppers, washed, seeded, and membranes removed	**1** Preheat oven to 350 degrees. Place the bell peppers in a baking dish and set aside.
1 cup dry lentils, rinsed and drained **2 cups low-sodium vegetable broth**	**2** In a medium pot, add the lentils and broth. Bring to a boil and then lower the heat; simmer for about 20 to 30 minutes and cover. Allow the lentils to absorb the liquid, stirring occasionally.
1 tablespoon extra-virgin olive oil **1 cup mushrooms, diced** **1 small shallot, diced** **1 garlic clove, diced** **2 sprigs fresh rosemary, coarsely chopped**	**3** In a small sauté pan over medium-low heat, add the oil, mushrooms, shallots, garlic, and rosemary. Stir together until heated through and the shallots are translucent. Add to the cooked lentils; gently stir. Pour in the tomatoes; mix well and add the paprika. Heat the mixture through. Remove from the heat.
One 15-ounce can fire-roasted tomatoes, undrained **1 tablespoon smoked paprika** **Parmesan cheese shavings (optional)**	**4** Spoon the mixture into each of the hollowed-out peppers. Place the peppers in the oven for 20 to 30 minutes or until the peppers begin to brown. Remove from the oven and top with shaved Parmesan (if desired). Serve immediately.

Per serving: Calories 362 (From Fat 61); Fat 7g (Saturated 1g); Cholesterol 0mg; Sodium 340mg; Carbohydrate 57g (Dietary Fiber 24g); Protein 23g.

Dishing Up Chicken and Turkey

In this section, I give you recipes that incorporate lean protein from poultry — namely, skinless chicken and turkey breast. Not only will you get good-quality protein, but you can make meals that are versatile and appealing to your whole family.

When cooking poultry, be sure to cook it to the right internal temperature: at least 165 degrees. Eyeballing your meat, especially with poultry, is not enough. Uncooked chicken and turkey poses a risk for *salmonella* poisoning; *salmonella* is a type of bacteria that can cause severe abdominal cramping, pain, and even death. You can't rely on color and texture alone to determine if your food is safely cooked. The only way to tell for sure whether your poultry has reached that key internal temperature is to use a good food thermometer. For handy tips on choosing, using, and cleaning a food thermometer, go to www.homefoodsafety.org/cook/food-thermometer.

Now let's get cooking! The great thing about poultry is that you can mix and match it with other food groups easily. You can easily add chicken or turkey breast to

- ✔ **Whole grains,** such as whole-grain pasta, brown rice, quinoa, whole-wheat couscous, and whole-grain breads, wraps, and pitas

- ✔ **Vegetables,** such as bell peppers, broccoli, carrots, cucumbers, mixed greens, onions, and snap peas

- ✔ **Fruits,** such as avocado, berries, grapes, kiwi, mango salsa, pineapple, and tomato salsa

- ✔ **Dairy products,** such as cheese (cheddar, mozzarella, provolone, Swiss), cottage cheese, and plain yogurt (for salad dressing)

If the idea of experimenting from scratch is a little intimidating to you, never fear: The recipes in this section will get you started!

Marvelous Turkey Meatballs with Balsamic Tomato Glaze

Prep time: 15 min • **Cook time:** 30 min • **Yield:** 4 servings

Ingredients	Directions
1 pound ground turkey breast, 93 percent lean	**1** Preheat the oven to 350 degrees.
¼ cup low-sodium Worcestershire sauce	**2** In a large bowl, add the ground turkey, Worcestershire sauce, bread crumbs, garlic powder, and onion. Mix to combine.
2 tablespoons whole-grain bread crumbs	
1 teaspoon garlic powder	**3** Using a small ice cream scoop, dollop a golf-ball-size round into your clean, washed hands. Massage into a ball. Repeat until you've used all the meat mixture (about 16 small meatballs).
1 teaspoon minced fresh onion	
1 tablespoon extra-virgin olive oil	**4** Place the meatballs in a nonstick pan over medium heat. Brown the outside and turn occasionally to get all sides of the meatballs. (To check doneness, use a food thermometer; the internal temperature should be at least 165 degrees.)
1 large garlic clove, minced	
3 Roma tomatoes, cored and diced	
1 tablespoon balsamic vinegar	**5** While the meatballs are in the oven, add the olive oil and garlic to a small saucepan over low-medium heat, and sauté for a few minutes until the garlic is translucent. Toss in the tomatoes and vinegar. Stir together until the glaze starts to thicken (or reduce). Remove from the heat.
Salt and pepper to taste	
	6 Add the meatballs to the glaze sauce and simmer for 5 minutes.

Per serving: Calories 240 (From Fat 118); Fat 13g (Saturated 3g); Cholesterol 84mg; Sodium 279mg; Carbohydrate 8g (Dietary Fiber 1g); Protein 22g.

Tip: Serve over whole-grain pasta or a bed of mixed greens.

Lemon Pepper Chicken

Prep time: 10 min • **Cook time:** 25 min • **Yield:** 2 servings

Ingredients	Directions
Two 5-ounce boneless, skinless chicken breasts	*1* Preheat the oven to 400 degrees.
1 medium lemon, juiced	*2* Place the chicken breasts in large plastic resealable bag. Add the lemon juice, pepper, garlic, and salt to the bag. Gently shake the bag to coat the chicken breasts with the lemon juice mixture. Set aside for 10 minutes.
1 teaspoon black pepper, ground	
1 clove garlic, minced	
Pinch of salt	*3* Place the chicken breasts with the juice mixture in a lightly greased baking dish. Bake for 15 minutes. Flip the chicken and cook an additional 10 minutes or until the juices run clear. (Use a food thermometer to verify that the chicken is cooked through; the internal temperature should reach at least 165 degrees.)

Per serving: Calories 167 (From Fat 33); Fat 4g (Saturated 1g); Cholesterol 91mg; Sodium 242mg; Carbohydrate 2g (Dietary Fiber 0g); Protein 30g.

Tip: A simple way to juice a lemon with a knife and fork only (no reamer needed) is to roll a room-temperature lemon on the countertop to pre-juice it. Then, using a sharp knife, halve the lemon lengthwise. Place a small strainer over a bowl to catch the pits, and squeeze each half of the lemon in your hand. Using a fork, scoop around to extract the additional juice.

Simple Turkey Burgers with Smokey Beet and Olive Relish

Prep time: 10 min • **Cook time:** 15 min • **Yield:** 4 servings

Ingredients	Directions
1 pound ground turkey breast, 93 percent lean	**1** Heat the grill. In a medium bowl, gently mix the turkey, mushrooms, half of the shallots, Worcestershire sauce, mustard, garlic powder, and cheese. When combined, use your hands to make 4 medium-size patties. Place on the hot grill. Flip the burgers once, cooking until the internal temperature is at least 165 degrees.
2 mushrooms, finely chopped	
1 medium shallot, minced	
2 tablespoons low-sodium Worcestershire sauce	
1 teaspoon Dijon mustard	**2** In the meantime, mix together the beets, olives, remaining shallots, oil, and paprika. Set aside.
1 teaspoon garlic powder	
2 tablespoons grated Parmesan cheese	**3** Dollop the burgers with the relish and serve.
1 cup precooked beets, chopped and mashed	
¼ cup black olives, diced	
1 tablespoon extra-virgin olive oil	
½ teaspoon smoked paprika	

Per serving: Calories 196 (From Fat 45); Fat 5g (Saturated 2g); Cholesterol 57mg; Sodium 283mg; Carbohydrate 6g (Dietary Fiber 1g); Protein 28g.

Tip: If you like, you can serve each burger on a plate with greens or on a whole-grain bun.

Simple Linguine and Chicken Puttanesca

Prep time: 15 min • **Cook time:** 20 min • **Yield:** 4 servings

Ingredients	Directions
One 13.2-ounce box linguine pasta 1 tablespoon extra-virgin olive oil 2 cloves garlic, minced Two 4-ounce chicken breasts, cut into small chunks 1 small shallot, minced 1 cup cherry tomatoes, halved ¼ cup Kalamata olives, chopped 2 teaspoons small capers, drained Pinch of black pepper Parmesan cheese shavings (optional)	**1** Fill a large stock pot with about 2 quarts of water, bring to a rolling boil, and add the pasta. Cook uncovered for 9 minutes, being careful not to over-cook. Drain well. Rinse in cool water to stop cooking, if desired. **2** Heat a small saucepan over medium-low heat. Add the oil, garlic, chicken, and shallots; sauté until the chicken is cooked through and golden brown. (To check doneness, pierce the thickest piece with a food thermometer to see if it has reached an internal temperature of at least 165 degrees.) Add the tomatoes, olives, capers, and pepper. Stir to combine and heat through. Bring to a simmer and remove from the heat. **3** Plate the pasta and pour the sauce on top. Sprinkle with cheese, if desired. Enjoy!

Per serving: Calories 449 (From Fat 59); Fat 7g (Saturated 1g); Cholesterol 36mg; Sodium 119mg; Carbohydrate 72g (Dietary Fiber 4g); Protein 25g.

Scrumptious Seafood

Eating from the ocean's bounty is not only healthy, but also offers a world of fabulous culinary options. Over the past couple of decades, nutrition science has shown that seafood offers a wealth of health benefits that may help to reduce the risk of heart disease, stroke, and cancer, as well as boost immunity. The cold-water dwellers, which contain a significant amount of omega-3 fatty acids, are the best options. Eat a variety of seafood to get your omega-3 fix.

The 2010 Dietary Guidelines for Americans recommends that the average adult get at least 8 ounces of seafood per week. For pregnant and breastfeeding women, at least 8 ounces and up to 12 ounces per week of a variety of seafood (but avoid high-mercury fish such as shark, swordfish, king mackerel, and tilefish and limit white albacore tuna to 6 ounces per week).

If you're allergic to seafood, you can take plant-based omega-3 supplements to get these beneficial fats. Or eat flax, chia, and hemp seeds, all of which contain omega-3 fats — aim for 2 tablespoons a day. As always, consult with your healthcare provider before taking any supplements.

What's the difference between seafood and fish? Seafood is the broad name for all marine life that live in the sea, as well as freshwater lakes and rivers. Seafood includes fish like salmon, halibut, tuna, tilapia, and trout, as well as shellfish like crabs, oysters, lobster, and shrimp.

A variety of seafood should be included in your diet because it offers good-quality protein and versatility to your overall eating pattern. Plus, you can have fun including a wide range of seafood into weekly dinners — whether grilled, baked, poached, or steamed. Enjoy making seafood in your kitchen with some of these simple and tasty recipes!

Broiled Maple Dijon Salmon

Prep time: 15 min • **Cook time:** 10 min • **Yield:** 2 servings

Ingredients	Directions
Two 4-ounce salmon filets	***1*** Preheat the broiler. Line a baking sheet with foil and lightly coat it with cooking spray or extra-virgin olive oil.
2 tablespoons pure maple syrup	
½ shallot, minced	***2*** Place the salmon filets on the baking sheet.
1½ teaspoons Dijon mustard	***3*** In a small bowl, stir the maple syrup, shallots, mustard, thyme, smoked paprika, and salt.
1 teaspoon dried thyme	
¼ teaspoon smoked paprika	
Pinch of salt	***4*** Brush the maple mixture over the salmon filets.
1 tablespoon minced flat leaf parsley	***5*** Place the baking sheet under the broiler and cook the filets approximately 10 minutes or to an internal temperature of 145 degrees. Be sure not to overcook, or the fish will be dry.
	6 Transfer the salmon to plates and garnish with parsley. Serve and enjoy!

Per serving: Calories 191 (From Fat 40); Fat 4g (Saturated 1g); Cholesterol 59mg; Sodium 155mg; Carbohydrate 14g (Dietary Fiber 0g); Protein 23g.

Lemon Halibut with Curry Dill Sauce

Prep time: 15 min • **Cook time:** 15 min • **Yield:** 2 servings

Ingredients	Directions
2 tablespoons extra-virgin olive oil	**1** Preheat the oven to 400 degrees. In a bowl, whisk the olive oil and lemon juice.
2 tablespoons lemon juice	
Two 6-ounce halibut filets	**2** Grease or spray a 9-x-9-inch baking dish. Place the halibut filets in the baking dish; season both sides of the filets with salt and pepper.
Pinch of salt and ground black pepper	
Curry Dill Sauce (see the following recipe)	**3** Drizzle the tops of the halibut evenly with the lemon mixture; rub gently. Set aside for 10 minutes.
	4 Bake the halibut in the oven for 12 to 16 minutes, or until it's easy to flake with a fork and opaque in color or the internal temperature is 145 degrees.
	5 Serve warm, topped with Curry Dill Sauce.

Curry Dill Sauce

⅓ cup nonfat plain Greek yogurt	In a bowl, mix the yogurt, mayonnaise, curry, garlic, and dill. Add the milk to a semi-thick consistency. Add the agave or honey and salt and pepper. Store in the refrigerator.
2 tablespoons light mayonnaise	
1 teaspoon curry powder	
1 clove garlic, minced	
1 tablespoon fresh dill, chopped	
2 teaspoons nonfat milk	
½ teaspoon agave nectar or honey	
Pinch of salt and ground black pepper	

Per serving: Calories 355 (From Fat 185); Fat 21g (Saturated 3g); Cholesterol 88mg; Sodium 348mg; Carbohydrate 7g (Dietary Fiber 0g); Protein 35g.

Sesame Shrimp and Broccoli with Angel Hair Pasta

Prep time: 10 min • **Cook time:** 10 min • **Yield:** 4 servings

Ingredients	Directions
8 ounces angel-hair pasta	*1* Cook the pasta according to the package directions; set aside.
1 cup broccoli florets	
2 tablespoons sesame oil	*2* Meanwhile, in a large sauté pan, place the broccoli, sesame oil, lemon juice, soy sauce, honey, scallions, and garlic. Bring to simmer over medium-low to low heat; cook 2 to 3 minutes, until the broccoli is crisp-tender. Add the shrimp; cover and cook 1 to 2 minutes.
¼ cup lemon juice	
2 tablespoons low-sodium soy sauce	
1 teaspoon honey	
1 small scallion, minced	*3* Divide the pasta evenly among individual bowls. Top with the shrimp and broccoli mixture. Sprinkle with sesame seeds, if desired. Serve warm.
1 clove garlic, minced	
1 pound large shrimp, peeled, deveined, and raw	
2 teaspoons sesame seeds, toasted (optional)	

Per serving: Calories 418 (From Fat 87); Fat 10g (Saturated 2g); Cholesterol 172mg; Sodium 446mg; Carbohydrate 50g (Dietary Fiber 3g); Protein 32g.

Tip: In this dish, feel free to substitute another type of seafood like crab, lobster, or salmon. The Asian flair of the sesame oil and soy sauce combination makes it a natural fit for seafood — fish or shellfish.

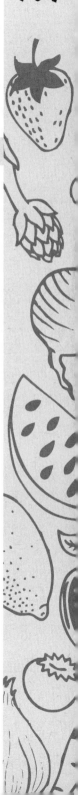

Got a hankering for red meat?

Good news: Any of the recipes in this chapter can be made with lean red meat. Yes, a steak or a juicy beef burger fits into your Total Body Diet plan! Keep in mind that spreading out your red meat consumption and choosing leaner cuts of meat with less saturated fat is important for keeping your heart healthy — as well as your weight in check.

Checking nutrition labels on red meat is important to determine the fat content in the meat. What is lean versus extra lean when it comes to cuts of beef? The U.S. Department of Agriculture (USDA) defines them as the following (in a 3.5-ounce serving):

✔ Lean meat contains less than 10 grams total fat, 4.5 grams saturated fat, and 95 mg cholesterol.

✔ Extra-lean meat contains 5 grams total fat, 2 grams saturated fat, and 95 mg cholesterol.

Go for leaner cuts of beef when you can for overall health. Look for the Choice or Select *not* Prime (because Prime is higher in fat — think prime rib).

Consider red meat as a side dish and stick with a smaller portion per meal — no more than 5½ to 6 ounces (1 to 2 servings) per day. Also, trim all visible fat like marbling from meat, drain the ground beef juices after cooking, and chill beef juices after cooking to skim off hardened fat. You can use the reduced fat beef broth as flavoring for rice, quinoa, stews, and soups.

Chapter 12

Desperts and Snacks

Americans love desserts and snacks! According to the Dietary Guidelines for Americans (2010), 35 percent of calories in the typical American diet comes from foods with solid fat and added sugars (think cookies and cakes), which adds up to about 800 calories per day. These foods take the place of more nourishing food sources, which contain essential vitamins, minerals, and dietary fiber. So, what's the solution? Limit and eat smaller portions of sweets and fat-laden snacks to make room for more nutrient-dense calories.

Sometimes a taste is all you need of a decadent chocolate dessert or a savory cheesecake, but creating options that allow you to get a bit more for the calories and ramping up the nutrient-density is ideal. You can have your cake and eat it, too — especially if it's made with good-quality ingredients like dark chocolate, whole-grain flour, and spices, and cut into smaller, single-serve pieces.

Here are some ways to shape up desserts and snacks:

✔ Add fiber with whole grains like whole wheat flour, oats, and nut flours.

✔ Toss in seeds — like flaxseeds, chia seeds, and hemp seeds — for heart-healthy fat.

✔ Whip in avocado for potassium and healthy fat for a smooth, satisfying texture.

✔ Sprinkle in flavorful phyto (plant) nutrients with spices like cinnamon, nutmeg, and cocoa powder.

✔ Use plant-based proteins like tofu, beans, and nuts to cut saturated fat from processed meats and full-fat dairy products.

✔ Mix in plain lowfat regular or Greek yogurt instead of sour cream or mayonnaise.

✔ Use fruits, fresh, frozen, or canned (in its own juice), as a natural sweetener instead of a lot of added sugar.

✔ Mix in peanut butter or almond butter for added flavor, texture, protein, and heart-healthy fat.

✔ Use fruit purees like apple, pear, or mango sauce instead of a lot of added oils or butter.

In this chapter, I give you some recipes for Total Body Diet snacks and desserts that can transform the way you snack, as well as end your meals in a better-for-you, sweet way.

Fruity and Sweet Treats

If you want a sweet fix, reach for fruit! Who doesn't love to bite into a juicy ripe peach, pear, or wedge of melon? Fruit is a delicious part of a healthy diet, and you should aim to eat at least 2 cups of fruit every day.

Whether you enjoy whole fruit as a handy snack on the go, or you prefer your fruit mixed with other ingredients as a tasty dessert, there's a lot of total body goodness that comes from fruit. Here are some of the health benefits of fruits:

✔ **It's heart healthy.** Fruit is free of cholesterol and saturated fat and it's virtually sodium free.

✔ **It's a natural blood pressure regulator.** Many fruits are loaded with potassium, the mineral that keeps blood pressure in a healthy range.

✔ **It's good for your waistline.** Fruit is low in calories and loaded with dietary fiber to fill you up longer and with fewer calories.

✔ **It's a potential cell health defender.** Fruit contains powerful antioxidants, such as vitamins A, C, and E, plus compounds called phytonutrients.

The latest research on antioxidants shows it's unclear whether it's the antioxidants in fruits (and vegetables) that contribute to good health or something else in these plant foods coupled with lifestyle and genetic factors that play a role.

✔ **It's hydrating.** Fruit is jam-packed with water and counts toward your fluid intake for the day.

Want to know what makes blueberries, blackberries, purple grapes, and raspberries so good for you? One reason may be that they all contain compounds called *flavonoids,* which are pigments present in blue, red, and purple fruits (and vegetables) that may help to reduce the risk of chronic diseases.

Some fruits are thought of as vegetables because their nutrition profiles, taste, and culinary purposes are more consistent with vegetables. Did you know that olives, tomatoes, and avocados are all fruits? Botanically speaking, they are. However, unlike other fruits, they're less sweet or tart, and they offer similar taste and nutrient content to other vegetables. Olives and avocados are jam-packed with monounsaturated fats, which are heart healthy. Plus, tomatoes are packed with a powerful carotenoid-antioxidant called lycopene. Research has shown that lycopene may reduce the risk of cancer — specifically, prostate cancer in men. Tomatoes eaten with a bit of fat like a drizzle of extra-virgin olive oil in marina sauce or a few slices of avocado in a tomato salad have shown to be particularly beneficial because the fat enhances the absorption of this fat-soluble nutrient, lycopene, in your body.

Honey Nut Apple and Citrus Gratin

Prep time: 20 min • **Cook time:** 20–30 min • **Yield:** 8 servings

Ingredients	Directions
6 apples, washed and thinly sliced	**1** Preheat the oven to 350 degrees.
3 tablespoons lemon juice	**2** In a large bowl, place the sliced apples. Add 1½ tablespoons of the lemon juice. Mix together.
2 tablespoons honey	
1 teaspoon cinnamon	**3** In a small bowl, combine the honey, the remaining 1½ tablespoons of lemon juice, the cinnamon, the vanilla, and the salt. Stir and add the chopped nuts.
1 teaspoon pure vanilla extract	
A pinch of salt	**4** Add the honey nut mixture to the apples and stir gently and thoroughly to coat all the apple slices.
⅔ cup walnut halves, roasted, cooled, and chopped	
Lowfat vanilla yogurt (for garnish)	**5** Place the apple slices into a 9-inch pie dish or individual ramekins and bake for 20 minutes. Check for bubbling and browning; if not done, place back in the oven for another 10 minutes. Remove from the oven and serve lukewarm with a dollop of lowfat vanilla yogurt. Enjoy!

Per serving: Calories 142 (From Fat 51); Fat 6g (Saturated 1g); Cholesterol 0mg; Sodium 21mg; Carbohydrate 25g (Dietary Fiber 4g); Protein 2g.

Strawberry, Coconut, and Blueberry Medley

Prep time: 10 min • **Yield:** 6 servings

Ingredients	Directions
3 cups strawberries, rinsed, hulled, and sliced	*1* In a medium bowl, gently toss together the strawberries, blueberries, and coconut.
3 cups blueberries, rinsed	
¼ cup coconut, flaked, unsweetened	*2* In a small bowl, squeeze the lemon halves until all the juice is captured. Add the honey to the lemon juice, and whisk gently until combined.
1 whole lemon, washed and halved	
1 tablespoon honey	*3* Drizzle the liquid mixture over the berries and coconut and gently toss again.
	4 Serve cold as a side dish or as a topping for yogurt or a slice of angel food cake.

Per serving: Calories 138 (From Fat 59); Fat 7g (Saturated 5g); Cholesterol 0mg; Sodium 5mg; Carbohydrate 21g (Dietary Fiber 5g); Protein 2g.

Tip: To hull a strawberry, take a small paring knife and carefully cut around the edge of the green leaves at the top of the berry. Cut in a circle and pop out the green inner stem. It will come out in a neat circular hole.

Cantaloupe, Basil, and Mozzarella Caprese

Prep time: 10 min • **Yield:** 4 servings

Ingredients	*Directions*
6 ounces fresh mozzarella cheese, cut into 6 medium-thick slices and then cut in half	**1** On a serving plate, place the mozzarella cheese rounds. Top each round with a cantaloupe slice and a basil leaf.
½ small cantaloupe, washed, halved, seeded, and sliced into bite-size pieces	**2** Drizzle with oil and vinegar and sprinkle with salt and pepper. Serve cold as a tasty snack.
12 fresh basil leaves, washed and dried	
1 tablespoon extra-virgin olive oil	
1 tablespoon balsamic vinegar	
A pinch of sea salt and black pepper	

Per serving: Calories 177 (From Fat 108); Fat 12g (Saturated 6g); Cholesterol 23mg; Sodium 272mg; Carbohydrate 6g (Dietary Fiber 0g); Protein 12g.

Mango Basil Salsa

Prep time: 10 min • **Yield:** 4 servings

Ingredients	Directions
2 large mangos, washed, peeled, pitted, and diced	*1* In a medium bowl, gently toss together all the ingredients.
1 small shallot, minced	
5 fresh basil leaves, washed, dried, and coarsely chopped	*2* Serve immediately on whole-grain crackers or pita chips or chill in the refrigerator for 15 minutes before serving. Store leftovers in the refrigerator for up to 3 days.
Whole-grain crackers or pita chips, for serving	

Per serving: Calories 69 (From Fat 3); Fat 0g (Saturated 0g); Cholesterol 0mg; Sodium 2mg; Carbohydrate 18g (Dietary Fiber 2g); Protein 1g.

Tip: To cut and peel a mango (after washing and drying it), simply take a sharp paring knife and peel off a thin layer of the skin. Then quarter the peeled mango by cutting to the pit or stone on the center and gently slice along the edge of the stone to remove the juicy yellow flesh. The stone likes to hang onto the flesh, so do your best to get most of it off.

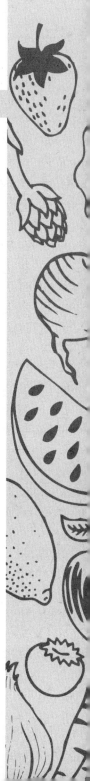

Chocolate Decadence

There's good reason to eat chocolate — and the darker the chocolate, the better! It's the cocoa powder — the part of the cocoa bean without the cocoa butter or solids — that contains the health benefits. Cocoa is rich in powerful antioxidants or a type of flavonoid called *flavanols,* which may benefit cardiovascular health by lowering blood pressure and helping to maintain normal blood flow.

The European Food Safety Authority approved a health claim for cocoa flavanols that states: "Cocoa flavanols help maintain the elasticity of blood vessels, which contributes to normal blood flow." The catch: You have to eat 200mg of cocoa flavanols to reap the cardiovascular rewards.

Be careful how you get the flavanols in chocolate, the calories can add up fast! Table 12-1 outlines the calories in various types of chocolate.

Table 12-1	Calories in Chocolate	
Ingredient	*Serving Size*	*Calories*
Cocoa powder	1¾ tablespoons	20
Baking chocolate	½ ounce	70
Semisweet chocolate	1½ ounces	200
Dark chocolate	2 ounces	320
Chocolate syrup	1 cup	840
Chocolate milk	10½ ounces	249

Source: Journal of Agricultural and Food Chemistry, *2009*

How the cocoa is delivered — whether in a bar or beverage — can impact your blood vessels. A recent study in the *Journal of Agricultural and Food Chemistry* found that cocoa flavanols in dark chocolate are eight times more effective at lowering blood pressure than a cocoa beverage with equal flavanols. Why? The researchers theorize that this may be due to the overall food medium (solid chocolate or diluted liquid) in which the cocoa is incorporated.

Just as choosing your chocolate wisely is important, so is savoring it. Use all your senses when eating chocolate to smell the scent of it, taste it on your tongue, and observe the feelings that a piece of chocolate evokes in your body when you swallow it. You'll enjoy a smaller amount, if you eat it mindfully.

Look for unsweetened cocoa powder — avoid *Dutch-processed* or *alkalized* cocoa powder, which means it's processed with a chemical to reduce the acidity of the cocoa. According to the USDA Nutrient Database, processing of cocoa powder results in a lower amount of flavanols.

Here are some tasty ways to add dark chocolate and cocoa to your day:

- ✔ Sprinkle cocoa powder into coffee and stir for an antioxidant-rich morning boost.

- ✔ Add a dash of cocoa powder to hot oatmeal or even over your favorite cold cereal.

- ✔ Toss a handful of dark chocolate chips into veggie and bean chili for hearty flavor.

- ✔ Melt a dark chocolate square and pour it into plain lowfat Greek yogurt and stir for homemade chocolate yogurt.

Dark Chocolate, Curry, Raisins, and Pistachio Bark

Prep time: 40 min • **Cook time:** 1 min • **Yield:** 12 servings

Ingredients	Directions
Two 8-ounce dark chocolate baking bars (at least 60% to 70% cocoa)	**1** Line an 8-x-8-inch baking dish with wax paper and set aside.
¼ cup raisins	**2** Melt the chocolate by placing it in a medium microwave-safe bowl and microwaving on high for 1 minute. Stir and put the bowl back into the microwave for another 30 seconds. Take out and stir the liquid chocolate. (You can also melt chocolate on the stovetop in a double boiler.)
¼ cup pistachios, lightly salted, coarsely chopped	
¼ teaspoon curry powder	**3** Stir in the raisins, pistachios, and curry powder. Spread into the prepared baking dish and put in the freezer for 15 to 30 minutes, until solid. Remove from the freezer and carefully chop the frozen block of bark into pieces with a large chef's knife.

Per serving: Calories 244 (From Fat 141); Fat 16g (Saturated 8g); Cholesterol 2mg; Sodium 4mg; Carbohydrate 23g (Dietary Fiber 3g); Protein 3g.

Salted Chocolate and Black Bean Brownie Bites

Prep time: 10 min • **Cook time:** 10 min • **Yield:** 9 servings

Ingredients	Directions
11 ounces dark chocolate (at least 60% to 70% cocoa)	*1* Preheat the oven to 350 degree. Line muffin tins with liners (or use nonstick muffin tins).
½ cup black beans, canned, rinsed, and drained	*2* In a blender or food processor, add beans and pulse a few times until pureed.
1 teaspoon pure vanilla extract	*3* Place the chocolate in a microwave-safe bowl and microwave on high for 1 minute. Remove the bowl from the microwave and stir. Put the bowl back in the microwave for another 20 to 30 seconds to melt if necessary. (You can also melt chocolate on stovetop in a double boiler.)
1 tablespoon agave nectar	
1 teaspoon cinnamon	
3 whole eggs	
⅔ cup self-rising flour	*4* Add the pureed beans to the melted chocolate. Stir in the vanilla and cinnamon. Crack the eggs into the mixture and fold in the flour. Gently mix together, being careful not to overmix.
½ teaspoon salt	
½ ounce semisweet chocolate for drizzling (optional)	*5* When combined spoon the mixture into muffin tins. Sprinkle with salt and place in the oven. Bake for 10 minutes or until a toothpick inserted in the center comes out clean. Remove from the oven and allow to cool for a few minutes. If desired, drizzle with melted semisweet chocolate for a bit of added sweetness. Enjoy!

Per serving: Calories 276 (From Fat 136); Fat 15g (Saturated 8g); Cholesterol 73mg; Sodium 324mg; Carbohydrate 29g (Dietary Fiber 4g); Protein 6g.

Dark Chocolate Dipped Berries and Pears

Prep time: 1 hr • **Yield:** 6 servings

Ingredients	Directions
1 cup dark chocolate (at least 60% to 70% cocoa), coarsely chopped	**1** Put the chocolate in a microwave-safe bowl and microwave on high for 1 minute. Remove and stir.
12 strawberries, stems removed	**2** Wash and dry the fruit well.
½ cup blueberries **1 ripe pear, sliced**	**3** Dip each piece of fruit into the chocolate individually. For the blueberries, use a toothpick to twirl them in the chocolate more easily. Drizzle chocolate on the pears, if they are too moist to dip into chocolate.
	4 Refrigerate the chocolate-dipped fruit for at least 30 to 45 minutes before serving or store in a covered container in the fridge up to 2 days. Enjoy!

Per serving: Calories 193 (From Fat 110); Fat 12g (Saturated 7g); Cholesterol 1mg; Sodium 6mg; Carbohydrate 19g (Dietary Fiber 5g); Protein 3g.

Yogurt Delights

Made from fermented milk, yogurt is teeming with *probiotics* (friendly bacteria), which are live microorganisms that offer your body health benefits. These armies of good bugs may help to combat the ill effects of disease-causing bacteria in your gastrointestinal tract and work to maintain good digestion and boost immunity.

Heat during processing can destroy probiotics in yogurt, so check yogurt containers and look for the words: *live and active cultures.* This refers to the live bacteria *Lactobacillus bulgaricus* and *Streptococcus thermophilus.*

The National Yogurt Association (www.aboutyogurt.com) created the Live & Active Culture seal to identify yogurt with at least 100 million cultures per gram at the time of manufacture.

Yogurt contains protein and calcium, but it can also be fortified with another bone-builder, vitamin D. Vitamin D is called the sunshine vitamin because your body makes vitamin D from sunlight. Only a handful of foods contain vitamin D, such as fatty fish like salmon and sardines, egg yolks, some cheeses, and white button mushrooms that are exposed to ultraviolet light. The average adult needs 600 international units (IU) per day; adults over 70 years of age need 800 IUs of vitamin D daily.

Want to get yogurt in your day? Here are some tasty ways to do it:

- Dollop a couple of tablespoons of plain, lowfat yogurt over a bowl of chili.

- Put a cup of plain lowfat yogurt in a blender with fruit and a tablespoon of nut butter to make a smoothie.

- Mix a tablespoon or two of plain, lowfat yogurt with Dijon mustard, dill, and a dash of white pepper and blend into tuna or diced cooked chicken breast for a savory salad.

- Crumble ¼ cup of lowfat granola, raisins, and a few dark chocolate chips over a cup of plain, lowfat Greek yogurt.

- Blend plain or vanilla lowfat yogurt with sliced strawberries and blueberries, pour into popsicle molds, and freeze for tasty hot-weather treats.

Crunchy Berry and Yogurt Parfaits

Prep time: 15 min • **Yield:** 6 servings

Ingredients	Directions
½ cup raw whole oats	**1** Toast the oats in a dry skillet of medium-high heat until golden brown.
6 cups plain lowfat yogurt	
2 cups blueberries, washed and dried	**2** In each of 6 fluted glasses, place ⅓ cup of plain yogurt. Add 1 tablespoon of blueberries, 1 tablespoon of oats, and a drizzle of honey. Repeat until each glass is filled to the top.
1 tablespoon honey	
1 teaspoon cinnamon	
6 sprigs fresh mint, washed and dried	**3** Top each glass with a sprinkle of cinnamon and a sprig of mint.
	4 Serve immediately or refrigerate until ready to serve.

Per serving: Calories 205 (From Fat 39); Fat 4g (Saturated 3g); Cholesterol 15mg; Sodium 172mg; Carbohydrate 28g (Dietary Fiber 1g); Protein 14g.

Vary It! Swap out the blueberries for any other berry of your choosing!

Frozen Yogurt Maple Nut Popsicles

Prep time: 15 min • **Yield:** 6 servings

Ingredients	Directions
4 cups plain lowfat yogurt	**1** In a medium bowl, mix together all the ingredients.
2 tablespoons pure maple syrup	**2** Spoon the mixture into six 6-ounce popsicle molds and put in the freezer for a couple of hours.
1 ounce almonds, coarsely chopped	
1 teaspoon pure vanilla extract	**3** Remove from the freezer and pop out of the molds. Enjoy a tasty frozen yogurt treat!

Per serving: Calories 150 (From Fat 45); Fat 5g (Saturated 2g); Cholesterol 10mg; Sodium 115mg; Carbohydrate 17g (Dietary Fiber 1g); Protein 10g.

Vary It! Nuts add a whole host of good things to this sweet treat. You can use an ounce of other nuts that you like. Any nut will add heart-healthy fats, fiber, and protein!

Ginger Spice and Raisin Yogurt

Prep time: 15 min • **Yield:** 4 servings

Ingredients	Directions
4 cups vanilla lowfat Greek yogurt	**1** In a medium bowl, mix together all the ingredients.
1 teaspoon fresh ginger, minced	**2** Spoon the mixture into small bowls and serve.
1 teaspoon nutmeg	
1 teaspoon cinnamon	
2 tablespoons raisins	

Per serving: Calories 191 (From Fat 0); Fat 0g (Saturated 0g); Cholesterol 8mg; Sodium 91mg; Carbohydrate 27g (Dietary Fiber 1g); Protein 20g.

Tip: Ginger has anti-inflammatory properties. Plus, it may help with nausea during pregnancy and after surgery. You can use it fresh from the root or dried and ground in powder form. Crystallized ginger is candied with a sugar coating — use it more sparingly because it contributes added sugar to the diet.

Part IV
Getting Mindful the Total Body Way

Five Ways Your Senses Can Lead to Good Health

- **Look at what you're eating.** How food *looks* is important. Appreciate the sights of foods and beverages. Notice the bold blue in blueberries or the bright red in cherry tomatoes or the deep green in peas. By taking the time to notice the shapes of your pasta and the jagged edges of your torn bit of crusty bread, you'll appreciate your eating experience more.

- **Listen to what you're eating.** Is your chicken sizzling on the grill? Is your popcorn popping on the stovetop? Is your coffee dripping in the pot? By noticing the sounds of cooking foods, you'll appreciate them with different depth. You can also determine doneness. When the popcorn stops popping, it's time to take it off the stove, and when the coffee stops dripping, it's ready to pour into a mug.

- **Savor and taste your food.** Many of the food choices you make are determined by taste, but are you really taking the time to taste what you eat? Slow down and savor the taste of smooth yogurt on your tongue or the spice in curried cauliflower or sour lemon on the baked chicken. As you focus on flavor, you'll chew more slowly and notice your fullness cues more easily, too.

- **Feel the texture of your food.** You probably aren't going to eat with your hands (unless the food requires it), but touching can happen on your tongue. If you hold an apple, orange, or potato in your hands, notice the weight and texture difference. Take the time to touch your raw vegetables, fruits, nuts, seeds, and grains. The tactile nature of touching food is important and cultivates an appreciation of its nourishing nature.

- **Bask in the aroma of nourishing food.** One of the most powerful senses as far as food is concerned is smell. There's nothing like the scent of fresh-baked bread or cookies. Embrace the aroma of your food by noticing its pleasant nature and how it whets your appetite with just a subtle waft when you enter the house or kitchen.

Get tips on eating a green diet — one that's good for the environment *and* for you — in a free article at www.dummies.com/extras/totalbodydiet.

In this part . . .

- ✔ Get into the mindful eating and living zone with skills, tactics, and techniques.

- ✔ Practice mindfulness by listening to your appetite and understanding what it's revealing to you.

- ✔ Make mindfulness part of every eating occasion — whether it's the holidays, a party, or a quiet meal for two.

- ✔ Turn cravings into real food moments by recording, savoring, and budgeting your calories wisely.

Chapter 13

The Ins and Outs of Mindful Eating

*B*eing mindful in our fast-paced society is counterintuitive — it seems like we have no time to stop and smell the roses. But mindful opportunities are everywhere, if you pay attention. Mindful-based practices have been around for centuries and modern science has shown mindfulness to be an effective tool for disease management, weight loss, and mood enhancement. Mindful eating is not a diet — it's a way to promote total body wellness that extends beyond the plate into your everyday life.

In this chapter, you get the comprehensive scoop on mindful eating and living and see where it can fit into your own life. I highlight the art of savoring your food, eating objectively without judgment, and getting to know your appetite. Did you know that you can get intimate with your appetite? Yes, you can (and will!).

Mindful Eating 101

With mindful eating, your world is your learning landscape. When you get the gist of it, you can be off and running! What I love about mindful eating is that you don't need to spend a lot of money on prepared meals and supplements or memorize a laundry list of rules and regulations or deprive yourself of foods that you enjoy. All you need is your mind and the desire to focus on the act of eating and all that it encompasses. As simple as it sounds, it can be a hard act to follow every day.

Imagine a world where you were only allowed to eat one food — you had no choices or variety. Day in and day out, you ate and drank the same thing. Not only would that be boring, but it wouldn't be nourishing for your body or spirit. Fortunately, we have a myriad of food choices every day. Research by Brian Wansink, PhD, author of *Mindless Eating: Why We Eat More Than We Think,* reports that the average person makes well over 200 decisions about food every day! So it behooves us to be mindful when choosing what, when, and how to eat.

Mindful-based practices have been around for centuries to alleviate stress, insomnia, overeating, depression, and many other health-related issues. By focusing on the positive, nurturing aspects of food, mindfulness allows you to foster a healthier relationship with food. You'll gain an understanding of what you're hungry for versus eating excess calories to fill an emotional void. Is it food or a hug you're seeking?

Mindful eating allows you to answer the following questions:

- ✔ Am I hungry for food, or is there some other reason I feel the urge to eat?
- ✔ Am I enjoying the food I'm eating?
- ✔ Am I savoring my food by eating slowly?
- ✔ Am I eating something that is nourishing and nurturing to my body?
- ✔ Am I satisfied after eating this meal or snack?

By being present in the moment and asking yourself these types of questions when you eat and make food choices, you'll build a greater intimacy with food — and you'll be healthier and happier, too. In the following section, I explain how to be more mindful with what you eat and drink.

Minding what goes into your mouth

There is no doubt that mindful eating takes practice. It's not easy to forgo the homemade cookie on your co-worker's desk or the last slice of pizza sitting in the box calling your name. Your mindful voice can get easily muffled among the chatter in your brain. Many times, instant gratification overrides mindfulness. How do you combat this? It's about shifting into the eating moment, according to Susan Albers, Psy.D., author of several mindful eating books, including *50 More Ways to Soothe Yourself Without Food.*

So, how do you get into the eating moment? Eating is fun and enjoying every moment of eating (and drinking) is a challenge. Taking time with the process is a large part of it. Think about how refreshing and soothing a glass of cold water tastes when you're hot and thirsty. If you pay attention to the cold sensation of the liquid on your tongue and then it hitting the back of your throat and plunging down your esophagus like a waterfall cooling you off internally, depositing into your stomach to aid in digestion, as well as hydration of every cell in your body, that gulp of water becomes magical! It takes on new meaning when you're in the moment. You begin to feel more fulfilled by the nourishing aspects of foods and beverages when your attention shifts there.

To get into the eating moment, stop and listen. If you're physically hungry and your stomach is rumbling, that's a sign to eat or drink. But if you just ate an hour ago and food looks appealing because you have a hungry heart and want to fill an emotional need or void, take a walk, take a bike ride, or call a friend.

Savor, savor, savor

One of the best things about mindful eating is that it's not about depriving yourself of your favorite foods. When I tell you that you can still have chocolate or potato chips or a hunk of crusty artisan bread with butter, do you read this in disbelief? It's true and it works! It's all about being satisfied on less — because your taste buds are actually programmed to enjoy less.

Research shows that taste buds are chemical sensors that tire quickly — the first few bites of a food taste better than the latter ones. After you eat a large amount, there is very little taste experience left at all. Which is precisely why it's important to savor and enjoy taking slow, deliberate bites to get the most satisfaction!

The primary driver of mindful eating is slowing down and savoring taste and flavor. As you move to a more mindful, slow eating place, you'll eat "from freedom instead of compulsion," as Michael Pollan explains in his book *In Defense of Food: An Eater's Manifesto.* "Eat slowly" is one of Pollan's eating tenets. He describes how slowing down your eating is about more than just the speed at which you eat; it cultivates knowledge for where food comes from, as well as gratitude for the bounty of nourishing food around us. Miracles unfold when you become a more mindful eater and savor food in a new way!

Looking in from the outside: The art of eating objectively

One of the best skills that comes from mindful eating is *objectivity* (basing perceptions on facts and logic instead of emotions and personal experience). You can stand and look at yourself from far away and determine your reactions to what and how to eat.

For example, you're dining out with friends and they order appetizers and you feel compelled to eat the fried calamari because it looks and smells delicious. You know from past experience that it tastes good, too! Let's explore how the art of eating objectively can come into play here. If you don't look at yourself from the outside in, you may wind up overeating mindlessly. You can look at it from afar in a couple of different ways (and neither one is right or wrong):

- ✔ Pass on the appetizer because you planned to eat an entrée and share a dessert — your plan prior to entering the restaurant.
- ✔ Take a small amount of calamari on your plate and savor it. Enjoy!

You can feel just as satisfied with either choice you make. Whether you stick with the plan you made prior to going into the restaurant or take a small amount and savor it (and decide to not have an alcoholic beverage or forgo bread or dessert). As a mindful eater, you have choices!

Every eating experience offers an opportunity to tap into yourself and trust your inner food guru. Step outside, look in, and view your available eating (and drinking) choices. It's liberating to be *nonjudgmental* with your choices by allowing all sorts of thoughts and emotions into your mind — the good, the bad, and the ugly. The goal is to notice the thoughts and not react to them. You don't have to give power to every thought you have. It's okay to "disobey the thought," as Susan Albers puts it in her book *Eat, Drink, and Be Mindful*.

Use the following examples to practice being nonjudgmental — it takes a lot of practice. Think about how you would talk to a friend — in a compassionate, kind way — and use that same tone with yourself.

Judgmental Thought (Black-and-White Thinking)	*Nonjudgmental Thought (Compassionate, Kind Thinking)*
My mother is overweight, so I always will be, too.	I am not my mother. I can control my weight.
I shouldn't eat this chocolate cake because I'm overweight and this will make it worse.	It's okay to have a small piece of the cake. I'll enjoy it and feel satisfied on less.
I can't wear shorts. My legs are stocky.	I prefer to wear skirts. They enhance my figure.
I can only eat organic apples. They're better for me and the environment.	If I can only find conventionally grown (nonorganic) apples, I'll rinse and scrub them well under cold water.
If I eat the full-fat ice cream, I'll blow my diet today and might as well eat whatever I want.	A small bowl of full-fat ice cream will satisfy me and keep me from overeating later (because I'll be full longer).
I feel bigger in my jeans after a night out of eating and drinking.	My jeans are a good gauge of my weight. I know to cut back if they're getting tight.

Developing Appetite Intimacy

So, you're beginning to understand that self-talk can help or hinder your mindful eating journey. You wouldn't be friends with a person who talks negatively about you or to you — so you shouldn't treat yourself that way either. Developing compassion and intimacy with yourself is important to total body wellness. This holds true for your appetite awareness, too. What is your appetite telling you? Are you listening to your hunger and fullness cues or can you not even hear them?

One of the first questions I ask my clients is: Do you feel hunger on a regular basis throughout the day? It's a good thing to feel hunger because it means your metabolism is working and your body is burning and churning through calories. If you don't feel hunger, it could be that you're ignoring it, your metabolism is sluggish, or you're eating so frequently that you don't get hungry.

Everyone has a different appetite — some people feel like they have an insatiable appetite, while others fill up fast regardless of their size and shape. The key with tuning into your appetite is listening to how hungry you are before you start eating and how full you are when you stop eating, according the *Appetite Awareness Workbook* by Linda Craighead, PhD. Discerning your appetite may be challenging at first, but it's based on your intuitive feelings, feelings that are unique to you.

Getting intimate with what I call your *tummy talk* (your stomach's rumbling and grumbling) is vital. Of course, there are other, less obvious signs of hunger:

- ✔ Lightheadedness
- ✔ Fatigue
- ✔ Nausea
- ✔ Headache
- ✔ Muscle weakness
- ✔ Low stamina
- ✔ Irritability
- ✔ Bad mood
- ✔ Poor concentration or lack of focus

Appetite awareness training, which encourages letting your stomach be your guide, encourages monitoring of appetite versus actual food and beverage consumption. Created by Linda Craighead, PhD, in the mid-1990s, appetite awareness training proved to be just as effective a treatment for eating issues (such as binge eating, reducing pre-occupation with food, and weight management) as any other treatment available.

What about the other side of the appetite coin, fullness? Discerning when you've had enough to eat may be easier, but getting past the point of fullness to that stuffed state is what you want to avoid (or lessen the incidence of), if possible. It takes 20 minutes for your brain to register that your stomach is full, which is another reason to eat slowly!

Look for the following signs of fullness (before you're stuffed):

- ✔ Slight sensations in your stomach
- ✔ Food no longer tasting as good
- ✔ Taking longer pauses between bites
- ✔ Finishing a portion-controlled plate of food (check in with yourself before you reach for seconds)
- ✔ A burp or two (in some cultures that's a compliment to the chef meaning you ate enough and are satisfied)

Are you really hungry for food?

Hunger can hit at random times in the day, but as you become more attuned to your appetite, you need to ask yourself if it's genuine physical hunger or whether you're just thirsty. When my two children were babies, it was fairly simple to ascertain physical hunger because they would cry, squirm, or start to root on my chest looking for breast milk. Many times, it made sense with their eating schedule, too. Now that they're in elementary school and have more autonomy (they can reach into the fridge or cabinet whenever they want for a snack or drink), when and what they're hungry for are two different things. If they're just hungry for something sweet — and didn't finish the majority of their dinner because they were "full" — that's not legitimate hunger. That's a craving. There's nothing wrong with cravings, but like Pavlov's dogs, if they get a sweet after every meal, they begin to crave it, even if they aren't *really* hungry. That's classical conditioning at its best!

Think about it, are you hungry at regular times of the day? Do you eat at regular times of day? My stomach unleashes hunger pangs at 7 a.m., noon, 3 p.m., and 6 p.m., like clockwork. I guess you can say that I've trained my hunger and appetite response. That's why it's helpful to stay on a schedule of eating and drinking — this way your body and mind expect to eat at certain times. Of course, sometimes your eating schedule can get derailed with work, school, family, and other commitments — and with all that comes emotional highs and lows. Many times, food becomes the scapegoat, the comfort zone, or safe haven in the turbulent sea of life, and listening to internal hunger cues goes out the window!

Your healthful eating pattern may get hijacked by *external cues* or signals that occur in your natural environment. Linda Craighead, PhD, author of *Appetite Awareness Workbook,* sites the following as the most common external eating cues:

- ✔ **Food:** When there's candy in the jar by your desk, you walk past it and take one.

- ✔ **People:** Your colleague is eating a dessert after lunch, so it cues you to eat one, too.

- ✔ **Places:** A hot dog and beer at the ball park. Need I say more?

- ✔ **Advertising:** Commercials can whet your appetite for a juicy steak or burger, even if you just ate.

Just because these external cues exist, that doesn't mean you have to give in to them and eat, if you aren't hungry. Knowledge that these cues exist is important because you have the freedom to think about the eating signal that's occurring and politely dismiss it.

I like to think of *internal cues* (signals that come from with you) as your little voice inside. You know, the one that says, "That piece of cake would taste so good, especially after losing the school election" or "I deserve that other glass of wine for getting through that stressful week." Here are the most common internal eating cues (which can be related to appetite or not):

- ✔ **Thoughts:** Your kids' macaroni and cheese looks so good (even after you ate lunch already).

- ✔ **Rules:** You tell yourself that you don't eat dessert during the week.

- ✔ **Beliefs:** Maybe you tell yourself that you can have an extra serving of pasta, if it's whole grain.

- ✔ **Feelings:** You feel terrible today, and you think ice cream will make it all better.

- ✔ **Physical sensations:** You feel a pit in your stomach after a breakup (which can lead to a hungry heart).

- ✔ **Routines or habits:** You eat when you're tired after a long day while relaxing in front of the TV. You may not even be hungry, but you eat mindlessly because you're destressing — and that's what you habitually do.

For true appetite awareness, according to appetite awareness training, it's important to get in touch with hunger and fullness cues — also called *internal appetite-based cues*. However, your body, mind, and spirit are sneaky — you may feel physical hunger, but it's a psychological hunger (for example, loneliness, sadness, anger, and so on) that can't be filled with eating or drinking. As you monitor your appetite, you'll get more in touch with your different hunger hankerings.

Appetite revelations: What your appetite is telling you

You can't go anywhere without your appetite, and the more you get in touch with what it's telling you, the better. You may be able tune out hunger pangs, especially if you're busy with work, school, or family obligations, but when you eat, your appetite comes back with a vengeance (because your body needs nutrients to live!). I encourage you to embrace physical hunger and understand where it's coming from and the ultimate reason for it.

It's easier to feed psychological hunger with food instead of addressing the underlying reasons. Food will never satisfy a hungry heart.

Your appetite — whether physical or psychological — is signifying a need for change. When biological hunger hits, it means your brain, blood, and other organs have churned through the available fuel and are in need of more nutrients to continue your day in a healthy way. So, you have to change your focus from whatever you're doing to make time for a meal or snack. For this reason, meal and snack times offer a reprieve in the day to savor, enjoy, and nourish your body and mind. Plus, you can accomplish tasks better when your appetite is satiated.

In a similar vein, psychological hunger is call to action or change. The trick is tuning into the need to make a change. You may be among the many people who lose their appetite when under stress, depressed, lonely, or tired. Or you may overeat to compensate for these feelings or procrastinate getting stuff done due to the psychological demands. Neither extreme is good — the former can cause unhealthy weight loss, and the latter can lead to overweight or obesity, which brings with it a whole host of other health problems.

Every day, make the following affirmations for success:

I am going to . . .

listen to my body and mind's hunger pangs.

try my best to discern between physical and psychological hunger.

eat and drink at regular times.

not eat when I am not hungry.

be kind to my body and mind's natural hunger.

consider my emotional ebbs and flows and not try to feed them right away.

Every time you eat or drink, keep a log of the time of day, your hunger rating on a scale of 1 to 10 (where 1 is famished and 10 is stuffed), how you felt before eating, and how you felt after eating. If you don't want to do this with paper and pencil, use your smartphone or computer. Just make sure to do it when you're eating — it's too hard to remember at the end of the day how hungry you were before you ate at 10 a.m.

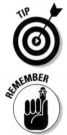

Jotting down your hunger rating may seem difficult in the beginning, but when you get the hang of it, you'll find that it works to assess your appetite before, during, and after eating and drinking.

Creating an appreciation for your changing appetite is a complex craft that takes time to master. Just as living the principles of the Total Body Diet is a continual practice that evolves over time, so does an appreciation for your unique appetite needs.

Your appetite fluctuates regularly — every meal brings a new appetite experience; each passing emotional tide shifts your appetite waves; and even your *circadian rhythms* (the way your body, mind, and behaviors respond to lightness and darkness over about a 24-hour cycle) affect your appetite. Think about dark and gloomy days when all you want to do is eat or the dog days of summer when food is not appealing at all.

Mindful Eating and Your Total Body Diet

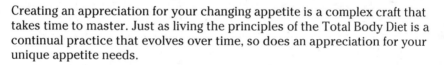

So, you may be asking, how does mindful eating connect to the Total Body Diet? In this section, I show you how to put your mind into eating. It takes practice. As Malcolm Gladwell describes in his book *Outliers: The Story of Success,* becoming a pro at anything takes at least 10,000 hours of practice. Amazingly, in every area of expertise from sports to music to writings to chess, this magic number of 10,000 hours of practice holds true. The reason noted in Gladwell's writing is that the brain requires this length of time to assimilate all that it needs to know to achieve true mastery. Even Mozart's concertos were not works of mastery until he logged in the hours!

That may seem like a lot of work, but the good news is that mindful eating can happen anytime, anywhere — soon, you'll be racking up the hours. In our seductive eating environment, where food is a constant temptation, you have an ideal landscape for becoming a mindful eating pro. Think about it: If you start today and practice mindful eating over the course of a year that's 12 hours awake most days times 365 days, or 4,380 hours of mindful eating and living!

The Total Body Diet is about making healthful, mindful choices *most of the time.* Yes, there will be times when you mindlessly munch or eat on autopilot because you've chosen to do that. The key is that the majority of the time you're aware of what, when, and why you're eating. Keep in mind that the more mindful eating you practice, the better you'll get at it.

Mindful eating, like anything else that you want to excel at, takes practice, practice, and more practice. Ten thousand hours is the magic number of greatness to adequately train your brain.

How to eat and drink mindfully every day

Start small on your mindful eating adventure. It always helps to not bite off more than you can chew (no pun intended!) when you start a new practice. Because this isn't a typical weight loss diet, but a mindful way of living. you don't even have to tell anyone that you're doing it. When you begin to change your attitude and put more mindful intentions forward, you'll see results begin to happen.

Here are some simple tricks to start practicing minding your eating and drinking today:

- ✔ **Give your body good food first.** Think healthy foods like vegetables, fruits, whole grains, beans, and lean protein before cake, cookies, candy, and chips. Eat nutrient-rich foods first and you'll have no room for other stuff.

- ✔ **Wake up with water.** After seven to nine hours of sleeping, hydrate your brain and body with an 8-ounce glass of water. This will not only wake up your brain, but it will also replace fluids lost overnight through your normal metabolic processes. And be sure to drink throughout the day because drinking water can help curb appetite.

✔ **Fill up on fiber.** Naturally found in plant foods, fiber is not digested in your body; instead, it imparts many health benefits, and can help promote a feeling of fullness, which can help with weight loss and maintenance. Strive for more fiber — women should ultimately aim for about 25 grams a day and men should aim for 38 grams. However, be sure to increase fiber gradually and drink plenty of fluids in the process to avoid distressing intestinal symptoms.

✔ **Eat and drink small.** Instead of thinking big, think small. Using small bowls, plates, and cups gives you the illusion that you're eating more than you really are.

✔ **Make time for tea.** Tea, especially green tea, is jam-packed with antioxidant compounds called *catechins,* which can defend your cells against free-radical damage. Sipping tea also helps you slow down, take a breath during the day, and alleviate stress. Plus, it displaces caloric beverages like soda, coffee drinks, and sports drinks.

✔ **Make a mental note every time you eat and drink.** Become more aware of everything you're eating and drinking. The goal is not to elicit guilt if you eat a cupcake, cookie, or French fries, but to create awareness around the quality and quantity of your calories.

The most important thing with mindful eating is to never feel shame, guilt, or anger toward your eating choices. Food is neither good nor bad — what matters is how much power you give it in your life. Mindful eaters don't label foods; they outweigh the positives and the negatives and choose to eat less of rich, high-calorie, fatty foods and more vegetables, fruits, lean proteins, beans, whole grains, and lowfat dairy products.

If you could follow a mindful eater and a mindless eater around for a day, here's what you would find:

Mindful eaters . . .	Mindless eaters . . .
Plan balanced meals and snacks to bring for the day ahead.	Pop into quick-service restaurants for breakfast, lunch, and snacks during the day.
Check the Nutrition Facts labels on foods for nutrient content as well as ingredients.	Don't read the Nutrition Facts labels, but may read what's on the front of the package, which doesn't give the whole story.
Eat sitting down and slowly.	Eat quickly while doing other things.
Find joy in cooking and creating healthful meals for them and their families and friends.	Don't enjoy cooking or find it challenging to put a healthful meal together.
Share meals and dessert when dining out.	Order large portions when dining out and don't always think to share.
Drink mostly water, tea, and coffee throughout the day, rarely a sugary, caloric beverage.	Drink whatever they want at the time, from sports drinks to energy drinks to gourmet coffees to soft drinks.

This gives you a snapshot into the opposing actions of being mindful versus mindless. This is not to say that sometimes the mindful eater doesn't fall into the mindless camp, and vice versa. Mindfulness is an art that has to be practiced over and over again. There's no perfect way — it's all about creating awareness around eating behaviors that you want to change, and sticking with it. Soon you'll see your total body respond with renewed health, vitality, and joy!

The benefits of mindful eating for your total body

There's a reason why mindful eating has stood the test of time. It's a kind, compassionate practice that welcomes everyone into the fold. Mindful eating experts contend that there's a higher degree of emotional intelligence that comes from minding your meals — and with that comes a healthier relationship with food. So you can temper emotional eating when you become more knowledgeable about how food choices affect your total body health and wellness.

I was struck by Dr. Susan Albers's concept called Eat. Q. No, it's not based on your IQ score, but there is intelligence that goes into it! In her book, *Eat.Q. Unlock the Weight-Loss Power of Emotional Intelligence,* Albers makes an outstanding case for Eat. Q., defined as aligning your intellectual knowledge of food and nutrition with your emotions, so you can make food choices that support your intentions and goals. Eating with intention is a mantra in many cultures — particularly in Buddhism where mindfulness was first established.

There's no doubt food is emotional — and it always will be as long as you have feelings associated with food. Think about it: There are foods you absolutely adore, foods you could take or leave, and foods that you flat out do not like. Taste preferences are part of the human, emotional condition — and research reveals that babies in their mothers' wombs have early taste experiences because flavors like cumin, garlic, and curry have been detected in the amniotic fluid of pregnant women. So, food preferences are established early!

Mindful eating is one of the tactics that I recommend you employ for total body wellness. Buy why? Mindful eating is a great prevention tactic — many areas of your body reap the rewards. From your cardiovascular system to your waistline to your blood sugar, mindful eating can come to the rescue.

Mindful eaters eat less, about 300 calories less a day — according to research in the *Journal of Nutrition Education and Behavior.* That can add up to gradual weight loss over time. Not only does weight loss come with mindfulness, but the science shows that it can help alleviate chronic diseases, anxiety, depression, and improve overall quality of life and well-being, which all bodes well for your total body!

TECHNICAL STUFF

The science behind mindfulness

Mindfulness, in the form of meditation, has shown to be an effective tool for managing disease states like diabetes. Anxiety and depression can ensue with a diabetes diagnosis and mindful meditative practices have been found to be helpful in transferring focus from the outside into the mind, brain, and body — the seats of the anxiety and depression. A randomized control trial in the *Journal of the Academy of Nutrition and Dietetics,* comparing a three-month group-based mindfulness-based eating awareness training for diabetes with a diabetes self-management education intervention in 27 and 25 people, respectively, ages 35 to 65, who had type 2 diabetes, non-insulin dependent, for more than a year revealed positive findings and a drive forward for future research this area.

In the mindfulness treatment group, participants engaged in guided mindfulness meditations, which involved feelings, experiences, and thoughts associated with food. There were no specific diet or physical activity goals set. They were encouraged to meditate at least six days a week — and do smaller or mini-meditations in between to create awareness of internal cues like hunger and stress, as well as outer cues, such as personal food knowledge and diabetes needs.

The other group received the goal-based behavioral program called Smart Choices. These participants were given total carbohydrate, calorie, and fat goals with an emphasis on food intake primarily.

In the end, comparison of the two groups showed reductions in weight and average blood sugar numbers called *hemoglobin A1C* (HA1C) in both groups. The researchers proposed that a mindfulness-based eating awareness training protocol, in conjunction with a goal-setting diabetes self-management education program, can be constructive for diabetes management. While both protocols offer different methods of treatment, people may do better if they can select which treatment or combination of treatments are most effective for them.

The good news is, mindful eating is receiving scientific recognition as an effective adjunct therapy to facilitate maintenance of lifestyle changes, which can be the most challenging part of diabetes management.

Getting hands on with mindfulness exercises

As a Total Body Diet enthusiast, there are many ways to get into the mindfulness mindset. It starts by using your body, mind, and senses differently. Mindful eating experts have discovered ways to slow down, savor, and sense your food better. Keep in mind, this all takes practice — and these exercises, although not very physical, are mental steps toward the mindful eating direction. If you practice them enough, you'll become a mindful eating pro.

Before you begin, ask yourself some questions:

- ✔ Can you switch hands when you eat?
- ✔ How can you focus on chewing more?
- ✔ Can you eat in silence without distractions?
- ✔ Can you taste the different flavors: sweet, salty, or spicy?
- ✔ What does the food smell like?
- ✔ What are the textures on your tongue?
- ✔ What is your posture like when you're eating?
- ✔ Are you open to try new foods and flavors?
- ✔ Can you take a smaller portion and savor it?
- ✔ What is the temperature of the food? Hot, cold, or room temperature?
- ✔ Are you enjoying this food or beverage? Why or why not?
- ✔ Is this a food you'd eat again? Why or why not?
- ✔ Does this food feel indulgent to consume? If so, why?
- ✔ Are you satisfied now that you're finished?
- ✔ How could this eating experience have been made better?
- ✔ Can you stop at half and take the rest home?
- ✔ How do you feel before, during, and after eating or drinking this?
- ✔ Would you brag to a friend about the taste and flavors of this meal?

It takes your brain 20 minutes to feel fullness. If you eat too fast and go back for seconds before your brain and body connect on the firsts, you'll have overeaten.

Now that you're getting your mind into you eating, how can you get your body into the mix by truly tasting better? Your tongue's taste buds sense five fabulous flavors: salty, sweet, sour, bitter, and umami.

Have you heard of umami? It's the fifth taste sense, and it's a Japanese word that means "savoriness." Foods that are high in umami are tomato products, dried mushrooms, Parmesan cheese, and anchovies.

Taste is one the tenets of the mindful, slow-eating approach and it's a fundamental part of good nutrition. It's no surprise that taste is cited as one of the most influential factors in food choice decisions. If you don't like how a food tastes, you aren't going to eat it. And no two tongues taste food the same way.

Your genes affect your ability to taste different flavors. According to the journal *Proceedings of Nutrition Society,* sweet and umami receptors help us discern carbohydrate and protein sources for energy, whereas bitter taste buds are highly sensitive and warn us of toxic foods entering the mouth — immediately your mouth's security system sounds. That explains why many children (and adults) gag at broccoli, Brussels sprouts, and kale on their plates.

Some people are blessed (or cursed) with the ability to sense taste with a far greater intensity than the average person; they're called *supertasters.* Supertasters typically taste bitter flavors more and don't like it. Research into supertasters and their food preferences shows that children and adults who have a heightened sense of taste are usually more discerning eaters.

I love doing this exercise with groups — I borrowed it from Susan Albers, Psy.D. All you need is a chocolate kiss or a mini chocolate candy bar. (You can do this with any food — it works well with a small cheese round, nuts, raisins, or sliced apples.) Follow these steps:

1. **Notice the weight of a piece of chocolate in your hand. Look at it closely.**

2. **Observe the shape and color. Use at least three words to describe it to yourself.**

3. **As you unwrap the piece of chocolate, listen closely to the crinkle of the foil or paper.**

4. **Bring the chocolate up to your nose, and inhale deeply. Notice what thoughts come in your mind as you do this. The smell of chocolate can bring up some powerful feelings and memories. Deeply inhale.**

5. **Do any critical thoughts come up like, "I shouldn't eat this"? If so, let the thoughts come and go as if you're letting go of a balloon.**

6. **Place the chocolate in your mouth. Notice the flavor, richness, and texture. Pay attention to how the sensations change as it melts and molds to your mouth.**

7. **Follow the sensations as the chocolate slips down your throat into your stomach.**

It takes practice eating chocolate . Notice how different this is from popping pieces of chocolate mindlessly into your mouth.

Mindfulness is an evolutionary process. Any moment can foster a new opportunity for mindfulness, if you allow it into your life.

Chapter 14

Mindful Eating for Every Occasion

· ·

In This Chapter

▶ Eating mindfully in various life situations

▶ Training your brain to be more mindful

▶ Building skills to conquer mindless eating

▶ Mastering mindful eating

· ·

Mindless eating opportunities are all around us. There's a candy dish at the dry cleaners, a platter of donuts and cookies tempting you at the office, free food samples at the grocery store, and indulgent snacks at your child's soccer game. The cards are stacked up high for mindful eaters — and especially for those in training. Mindful eating and living requires practice, patience, and resilience. Perfection is not possible, but striving to do better is.

When you've embarked on the journey of mindful eating, every eating opportunity becomes a chance to craft your skills. You'll lose the fear that comes from daily eating decisions — and make them joyfully, objectively, and without judgment.

In this chapter, you learn how to go into different eating decisions with the knowledge of internal hunger of when to start and when to stop eating. You'll learn to eat with intention and gratitude for the food on your plate, as well as respect where and how it was made and grown.

Making Sure You're Never Caught Off Guard

It's easy to get caught off guard with food popping up everywhere. That's why you want to wake up in the morning with a mindful eating mindset. By starting the day with a game plan — consisting of structured meals and snacks — and envisioning what the day's events may bring, you'll make mindfulness part of your everyday life.

Here are some simple ways to put on your mindful eating cap:

- ✔ **Before your feet hit the floor in the morning say a *mindful eating mantra* (a simple phrase or sentence to keep you present in the moment of eating).** For example, your mantra can be as simple as, "I am going to be present with my eating today" or "Tune in today." By saying your mantra a few times before you get out of bed, it's more likely to stick with you.

- ✔ **If you have a setback, realign yourself right away.** There's no reason to fret about a cookie at work or cheese ravioli sample at the grocery store, but getting back on the right eating track is essential. Knowing what and when you've eaten is vital to building a mindful, long-term relationship with food.

- ✔ **Plan balanced meals and snacks so that you don't mindlessly munch throughout day.** According to the book *Mindless Eating: Why We Eat More Than We Think,* by Brian Wansink, PhD, we have an "imperfect food memory," and our stomachs are bad at counting calories, especially when we've wolfed down a bag of chips at the kitchen sink or eaten ice cream while watching our favorite TV shows. The solution is planning — the more structure to your eating, the less apt you'll be to stray.

In the following sections, I offer tips on how to maintain your mindfulness no matter where life takes you — from vacations to holidays to parties to weekends.

Holding onto common sense on vacation

Time off from work to relax is a basic human need. It's easy to throw in the eating towel when you're traipsing around Europe or relaxing by a lake or at the beach. With delicious culinary choices and friends and family around, there's more opportunity to eat and drink. There's nothing wrong with that as long as you do it in a mindful way.

Planning your vacation time may seem counterintuitive. You want to go into your week away with looser reigns, but still keeping an eye on what I call your *mindful eating compass* — the inner sense or guide of what and how you're eating. If your mindful eating compass is steering away from healthful foods like vegetables, fruits, lean proteins, beans, nuts, lowfat/fat-free dairy products, steer it back on course at the next meal or snack. Keep in mind, it's not all or nothing — you have the freedom to make mindful food choices, even when you're on vacation.

Here are some simple tips to reining in your eating while on vacation:

- ✔ **Pack healthy snacks like whole fruits, nuts, whole-grain crackers, rice cakes, or trail mix on your vacation adventures.**

- ✔ **Stay hydrated with water.** It's tempting to drink more alcohol than you would normally, but alcohol can dehydrate you — and it packs a lot of excess calories. You can cut calories in alcoholic beverages by adding sparkling water to wine for spritzers or a splash of 100 percent fruit juice and cut-up fruit for a mocktail.

- ✔ **Don't skip meals.** If you do, you'll be ravenous and overeat foods that may not be the healthiest.

- ✔ **Eat the foods you like, but just in smaller portions.** If there are chips and guacamole or bread and butter on the table at a meal, put a small portion on a plate and eat that instead of grazing mindlessly. For dessert, choose a small sweet treat like a brownie square or a cookie. Savor and enjoy!

Keeping your head over the holidays

Mindful eating is tough around the holidays where socializing and food are closely linked. The holidays are notorious for weight gain, but recent research in the journal *Physiology and Behavior* reveals that the average American gains about one pound between November and January. That doesn't seem like a lot, but over time that one pound a year of weight gain adds up. How can you keep your mind in the eating game when the season to eat and drink is upon you? Modifying your behaviors, especially at this time, can help fend off weight gain while still allowing you to enjoy all the fun of the season.

With family, social, and work gatherings a big part of the holidays, setting boundaries will enable more mindful eating at this time. Here are some ways you can make mindful eating a priority over the holiday season:

- ✔ **Maintain your food, feelings, and physical activity logs.** You'll be more aware of the holiday extras that creep in, as well as the emotions that come into play with your eating events.

- ✔ **Don't give up your regular physical activity.** Fitness fuels eating well and vice versa. Squeeze in your workouts where you have to, if time is tight.

- ✔ **Be choosey about which events you attend.** It's okay to decline, politely — steering away from some events will keep you on your schedule of healthy eating.

✔ **Savor the power of one.** Don't deny yourself your aunt's holiday cookies or your brother's famous truffle candies — take one and savor it. Think about the taste of it in your mouth, on your tongue, and seeping into your taste buds as you swallow it. Truly enjoy *that* one.

✔ **Evolve your eating.** Think about the bounty of good food that you're fortunate to have access to, such as fruits, vegetables, whole grains, beans, nuts, seeds, eggs, lean meat, poultry, fish, and lowfat dairy foods. Evolve how and what you eat — your holidays will be more enjoyable for it!

Planning before the party

Who doesn't love a good party? Whether it's a birthday, engagement, retirement, wedding, or graduation party, eating and drinking are part of the fun. Whether you're the partygoer or party thrower, it takes planning. Either role takes a good dose of mindfulness to balance your consumption before, during, and after the event.

Here's a party planner checklist for the party thrower and the partygoer to create a mindful event:

Party Thrower	*Partygoer*
Don't throw the party hungry. Eat regular meals (and avoid snacking on party food during the setup).	Don't go to the party hungry. Eat regular meals and a snack within an hour of the party to satisfy hunger.
Plan healthy food options for guests like veggie platters and hummus, steamed spring rolls, salads, chili, soups, grilled meat, and chicken and veggie kabobs.	Circulate the room and don't hang out by the food table. Instead, peruse the options, take a plate of food, sit down, and enjoy.
Hydrate with water before the party. Drink alcohol moderately. For overall health, it's smart to drink responsibly — one drink for women and up to two drinks for men. (The more you drink, the more likely you are to mindlessly eat.)	Hydrate with water before the party. Drink alcohol moderately. For overall health, it's smart to drink responsibly — one drink for women and up to two drinks for men. (The more you drink, the more likely you are to mindlessly eat.)
Exercise the day of the party to alleviate stress and keep your energy up during the party.	Exercise before the party to offset additional calories that you may consume.
Relax and enjoy your guests!	Enjoy the company and not just the food!

Waking up to healthy eating on weekends

You know the drill: You're so on top of your eating during the week — keeping neat and tidy food logs; planning healthy, balanced meals and snacks; drinking plenty of water and limiting sugary beverages, alcohol, and highly processed foods. And then Friday night and it all comes loose. What's the deal with weekends? So much is tearing you away from your mindful eating mantra: You sleep later, do more social eating (and drinking), and have less structured time and, thus, less planning.

Mindless weekends can easily lead to weight gain and stop weight loss, according to a study in the journal *Obesity,* which included 48 healthy adults, ages 50 to 60 years, comparing one year of calorie restriction and one year of daily exercise. The results showed that both groups were down in calorie balance on weekdays, but it was a different story on weekends. Both groups consumed more on the weekends and were less active, which halted weight loss in the calorie restriction group and lead to weight gain in the daily exercise groups. These results make the case for mindfulness on the weekends.

Get mindful on the weekends in the following ways:

- ✔ **Start weekends in a healthy way with a balanced breakfast.** Try these:
    - Oatmeal, lowfat milk, and berries
    - Whole-grain toast, a scrambled egg, and a sliced tomato
    - Whole-grain cereal, plain lowfat yogurt, and sliced fruit
    - A banana, berries, flaxseed, and kefir smoothie

- ✔ **Get enough sleep, but not too much.** Catching up on sleep on the weekends sounds like a good idea, but the reality is that more than nine hours of sleep a night just throws off your day. Stay on track by setting an alarm on weekends. Indulge yourself in bed by hitting snooze a few times for a few additional minutes of shut-eye, but get excited for the day ahead. You'll feel better for it!

- ✔ **Get moving.** Plan physical activity into your weekends. You don't have to go to the gym, but you can walk to or from the store, take your kids to the park, walk your dog, take a bike ride — whatever you want and like to do, go for it.

- ✔ **Plan to eat one meal out, but the rest in.** It's okay to eat out on weekends, just not every meal. Typical restaurant meals add up to excess calories, salt, and sugar. If you limit the dining out on weekends, you'll save calories and money, too.

A Mindful Eating Toolbox for Total Body Wellness

There are a bevy of mindful eating tools that you can use in your everyday life for total body wellness — the key is knowing what they are and how to make them work in your life. Let's look at things that you can throw in your mindful eating toolbox.

With the focus on building a healthy relationship with food and fostering long-term healthy eating habits, the Total Body Diet aims to teach you new ways to talk to yourself about food, soothe yourself without food, and recognize *and* tackle the emotional eating triggers that cause overeating by listening to your *inner food guru* — that little voice that tells you if you're hungry or full.

Talking the mindful eating lingo

Have you ever thought about how you talk to yourself about food? Called *mindful speech* by Dr. Susan Albers in her book *Eat, Drink, and Be Mindful,* it's a compassionate, empathetic, and kind way to talk to yourself. It may sound simple, but changing your lingo to muffle the critical self-talk that has seeped in over the years takes constant practice. With how and what you eat, what you say inside can set the tone for your day and overall life!

Mindful eating lingo that's kind and compassionate sounds like this:

- ✔ "I don't have to be perfect. I just need to keep trying."
- ✔ "What I choose to eat is my personal decision."
- ✔ "If I were one my friends, I'd forgive myself and move on."
- ✔ "I need to pause, take a breath, and center myself again."

Fill in the sentences below to practice your compassionate mindful lingo in your whole life:

I am a good person because _____.

My greatest talent is _____.

My friends would say I am _____.

I am proud that I _____.

Rewarding yourself without food

As you work on your mindful lingo with food, as well as your total body wellness, think about ways to pat yourself on the back when you've come through an eating challenge or worked hard to let go of old ways and forge new pathways. Small steps deserve praise and recognition — even if only in your mind. Picturing your goals in your mind's eye and then a non-food reward once you've achieved it (for example, a new dress, diary, or book to read). Research has shown that children respond to nonfood rewards, such as stickers and verbal praise, and choose healthier foods as a result. Also, when you have something to look forward to, it makes day-to-day life happier!

Set up a monthly goal calendar and write in rewards to look ahead for. Here's an example:

Week	Goal	Reward
1	Incorporate veggies at snack time daily.	Get a manicure or massage.
2	Bring lunch to work daily.	Go to the movies.
3	Eat fish at least twice this week.	Get a new book.
4	Have an ounce of nuts (almonds, walnuts, pistachios) every day this week.	Buy a new water bottle.

Here are some other ways to reward yourself besides eating and drinking:

- Getting a facial or a haircut
- Buying new clothes, shoes, or makeup
- Buying kitchen gadgets or culinary tools
- Taking a day trip to a nearby town
- Buying walking or running shoes
- Signing up for a 5K race
- Buying tickets to a musical, play, or opera
- Downloading new music
- Planning a vacation to visit friends or family

Saying farewell to emotional triggers

Feelings — both positive and negative ones — are naturally connected to food. Think of the foods that make you happy. They could remind you of social gatherings, holidays, or dishes your grandmother made with love. As a mindful eater, it's great to identify with these feelings and appreciate them — and then step aside, allowing the nourishing aspect of foods to take the lead. For example, you love your grandmother's shoestring fries and steak. It not only tastes good, but it offers your body vitamin C and potassium in the potatoes and protein and iron in the steak. But it's not a good idea to eat this meal every week due to its high dose of saturated fat. So, when you do have it, relish the flavors, aromas, and positive feelings it evokes.

What do you do when certain foods are *emotional triggers* (foods that cause you to overeat for other reasons besides hunger)? Positive emotions (like happiness, contentment, and joy), as well as negative emotions (such as loneliness, sorrow, and anger), can cause you to eat — and potentially overeat. There's nothing wrong with an occasional chocolate or potato chip indulgence, but when it becomes a regular occurrence, there may be an issue.

If you want to rid yourself of emotional food triggers, look at your food choices differently. The operative word is *choice.* You have the power to choose to eat that food or not. Instead of putting the power on the food or beverage, take back the power to choose. In her book, *Eat.Q.: Unlock the Weight Loss Power of Emotional Intelligence,* Susan Albers, PsyD, points out that subtle words like *can't, should, ought to,* and *must* drive you to want craved foods more. Think about it: If you say, "I can't have chocolate," it takes away your power to choose and you want the forbidden chocolate. But if you say, "I choose not to have chocolate now," it's not a permanent directive — it's more flexible, which enables you to maybe have some later, or not. Find words that are empowering rather than victimizing when it comes to food.

If you're feeling emotionally powerless with food, seek advice from your primary care physician, a mental health professional, or a registered dietitian nutritionist (RDN) who specializes in eating disorders.

Saying Goodbye to Saboteurs

Your environment is a complex place filled with people, places, and things that can sabotage your efforts for total body wellness. It's easy to shed saboteurs, if you have a mindful mindset.

Dining out smart

Many restaurants have websites where they list current menu items, nutrition information, and recipes. A myriad of websites are devoted to restaurant nutrition information. For example, check out www.healthydiningfinder.com.

Here's a checklist of ways to be a mindful eater when you dine out:

✔ Avoid the "get your money's worth" buffet syndrome.

✔ Don't go to the restaurant ravenous.

✔ Look at everything on the menu before making your choices.

✔ Downsize — don't super-size.

✔ Incorporate low-calorie and filling vegetables.

✔ Ask for bread or chips to be removed or not brought to the table.

✔ Share desserts with others.

✔ Always ask for sauces, gravies, and dressings on the side and use them sparingly.

✔ Ask the waiter to hold the cheese or go easy on the cheese.

✔ Avoid menu items that are fried, crispy, creamed, au gratin, breaded, or scalloped.

✔ Reduce the mayonnaise, nuts, bacon, sour cream, butter, guacamole, and other high-fat condiments.

✔ Watch out for liquid calories (alcoholic beverages, regular sodas, and juices).

✔ Eat slowly. Chew your food carefully and put your utensils down between bites.

✔ Stick with lean cuts of meat, such as fish, chicken, turkey, bison, beef, or pork tenderloin.

✔ Ask for a to-go box when the food is served. Then put half of what's on your plate into the box — before you start eating.

Restaurant menus are designed to lure you into ordering foods that you imagine will taste good for a higher price, according to research by Brian Wansink, PhD, author of *Slim by Design: Mindless Eating Solutions for Everyday Life*. It doesn't hurt to ask the wait staff for lighter menu items that get the most raves.

Creating a new work environment

Whether you're a new hire or a tried-and-true employee where you work, you can always change up your work environment to a more mindful eating space. One of the biggest complaints I hear when I see weight loss clients is that co-workers are bringing in unhealthy treats and filling up candy dishes to tempt the office. You can be the beacon of change in your workplace by instigating new mindful eating rules of conduct (if for no else, but yourself!).

Mindful eating rules of conduct at work might include the following:

- ✔ Choose fruits, vegetables, nuts, seeds, and lowfat yogurt as snacks at work.

- ✔ Limit dining out by bringing a healthy, balanced lunch to work. Sit and eat it away from your computer or phone.

- ✔ Eat a snack midafternoon (around 3 or 4 p.m.) to avoid getting too hungry before dinner and stopping off on the way home from work.

- ✔ Sip water (still or sparkling) throughout the day. Limit your soda (regular and diet), gourmet coffee drinks, and juices.

- ✔ If possible, take a different route to the bathroom, boss's office, or exit if you have to pass the candy dish, vending machine, or cafeteria. Or replace the temptations with a fruit bowl and get the whole office eating healthier.

- ✔ Seek out an accountability partner. By asking someone else to join in your efforts, you can set goals together and follow up with each other.

When healthy foods are more convenient, attractive, and normal to consume, you're more apt to eat those foods. In the journal *Psychology and Marketing*, a study found that when foods are placed in a convenient place on the counter in attractive packaging and its normal to eat (like produce in front of the fridge or on the counter), it was eaten more often!

Making healthier convenient choices

As mentioned earlier in this chapter, if healthy foods are convenient, you're more apt to eat them. Society is plagued by unhealthy convenience foods, so how do you make healthier foods easier to access? There are key ways to make healthier foods top of mind. Sometimes even the most mindful eaters can miss the healthier options, if they aren't apparent or a more enticing food catches their eye first.

Here are some surefire ways to make healthier foods more convenient:

- ✔ **At home:** On the center of the counter, put a fruit bowl. In the center of the fridge, place cut-up veggies, lowfat yogurt, and kefir and fruit squeezes and ground flaxseeds.

> ✔ **At the office:** Put a fruit bowl at the reception area. In the kitchen, stock healthy snacks like nuts, yogurt, and fruit.
>
> ✔ **On the go:** Bring fruit, homemade trail mix (almonds/walnuts, raisins, and lowfat granola), and baggies of popcorn or rice cakes.

Craving Healthful Foods First

Some foods are hard to resist. Why are food *cravings* (intense desires for a specific food that is difficult to resist) associated with three key ingredients: sugar, salt, and fat? These flavor sensations activate the reward centers of the brain, according to the book *The End of Overeating,* by David Kessler, MD. Craved foods like cake, pizza, and fried foods activate pathways in the brain to want more of that food while it's being eaten.

Food cravings among overweight and obese people have been studied using a tool called the Food Craving Inventory (FCI), which is made up of 28 food items and ranks the frequency of the cravings, which are self-reported by research subjects. With everything from chocolate, which scores high in the list, to pasta to hot dogs to candy, craved foods run the gamut in the sugary, salty, fatty realm. And people with a healthy body weight have food cravings, too, because the brain is set up to desire these highly palatable foods.

Instead of fighting unhealthy food cravings, you can thwart the cravings with some good-for-you swaps. Imagine an intense desire for rice cakes and hummus or pistachio-crusted baked chicken breast or roasted vegetables and quinoa. By retraining your palate to want less sugar, salt, and fat, you'll soon discover that your cravings will start to turn that way.

Turning food cravings into healthy food moments

The whole gist of eating with intention toward health, happiness, and inner peace falls in line with transforming your cravings into healthy foods moments. Stopping to ask yourself some real questions while in the throes of a food craving is vital. What if you could trick your brain into wanting more healthy foods by making them delicious to your senses? Thinking on your feet to make healthy food swaps can be challenging, but it's effective.

Here are some food craving swaps to add more filling vegetables, fiber, whole grains, and healthy fats:

Food Craving	*More Healthy Craving*
French fries	Baked sweet potato fries
Pepperoni pizza	Veggie pizza with whole-grain crust
Linguini alfredo	Angel-hair pasta with pink tomato sauce (made with part-skim ricotta cheese)
Chocolate cake	Dark chocolate cake pop
Bacon cheeseburger	Turkey burger with avocado, lettuce, and tomato

Allowing small indulgences and moving on

It's difficult to swap every one of your cravings. The key is to put a halt on giving in to them too much. If you don't, your whole body will feel the overindulgence — and over time it will lead to excess inches, pounds, and potential health risks. However, savoring small cravings, like an ounce of dark chocolate or ½ cup of ice cream or a mini-burger, puts the craving in its place — as a smaller part of your world.

Mastering the art of small indulgence is truly a craft that you have to hone and develop over time. It does work — as your mind and body become more aligned to what you need. As much as you need to make room for healthful foods, you need to leave space for a few indulgences. Relegate the sweets and treats for a small part of your caloric intake because they take up prime nutrition real estate that more quality calories could be occupying.

Here's how to allow room for small indulgences:

✔ Practice taking smaller bites of cake, cookies, candy, chips, and fries. The smaller your bites, the more you'll savor it and enjoy eating less.

✔ Share desserts with others.

✔ Pair fruit with a drizzle of chocolate, such as pears or strawberries. You still get your chocolate fix, but in a small dose.

Writing it down

I have a client who emails me her food logs every night. It's a simple act with no bells or whistles. It's just the food and then a sentence or sometimes just a phrase about her feelings for the day. She finds solace in writing it down.

Picture reading your food diary five years from now. You'll see how far you've come with your emotions, feelings, and relationship with food. It's insightful and empowering to see your progress. Not only does the act of writing help you in the present, but it sets a tone for the future. It allows you to look back and realize how far you've come.

Every day, set the intention of at least writing down a thought, feeling, or association between food and you. It could be any of the following:

- ✔ What and how you ate at your meals (for example, "Moderate plate of pasta with clam sauce in record speed — rushing to get to the theater")

- ✔ Why you ate what you ate (for example, "Hot fudge sundae at a kid's birthday party")

- ✔ Emotional triggers that day that lead you to overeat (for example, "I was on a tight work deadline so I ate an entire bag of salt and vinegar chips at my computer; didn't feel great about that choice later, but it didn't define my day")

Now grab a notebook, scrap of paper, or your smartphone and jot it down. If you write it down, you won't forget it — and chances are, you'll learn a thing or two about yourself!

Budgeting for Extras

As part of your calorie accounting measures, your Total Body Diet ledger should factor in extras — like an ounce of dark chocolate or a few crackers with an ounce of cheese or a small vanilla latte. Your energy balance (calories in versus calories out) won't be thrown off if you factor in extras along with moving more. The key is to do it mindfully and know going in that you have to eat slowly and savor what you eat.

If you gulp down your food without chewing enough, it's almost like it never happened. So chew consciously and thoroughly. You'll enjoy it more!

Choosing healthful foods and less (unhealthy) extras

It makes you feel better to know that you can have a couple of small extras every day. However, factor in that pudding cup *after* you've had plenty of nutrient-dense foods. Ask yourself, "Have I had fruits and veggies today?"

Consciously make a decision to eat those foods first. You almost crowd out the unhealthy choices with the healthy stuff.

Try not to make a loaded extras decisions first thing in the morning. Instead, enjoy a healthy breakfast of a slice of whole-grain toast with a tablespoon of peanut butter and a small piece of fruit or a cup of whole-grain cereal with lowfat milk and berries. Typically, you know you'll want an extra fix after lunch or after dinner, so wait and make the decision based on the nutrient-density of your food choices overall that day.

Budgeting your calories (with your finances)

If it was as easy to burn through calories as money, waistline watching would be a breeze! One of the greatest ways to look at your calories budget is like your financial budget. It's like balancing your checkbook. Do you think hard when you spend $100 extra a day or do you just do it, record it in your check ledger, and know you have X amount of money left to spend? Like extra money in the bank — saved for a rainy day — saving calories provides you with the security of not overdrawing your energy account and allows you more to spend (or expend — as in physical activity) later. It's a balancing act that provides stability, as in body weight and fiscal status.

For example, say you spend 300 extra calories today on a candy bar. Could you have saved those calories or even spent less by forgoing the candy bar or having a mini candy bar instead? Balance comes in with expending the extra calories. So, if you know you're going to run two miles or bike to and from work and burn those extra calories, then go for it! But if you're just sitting around, the extra calories may pack on extra pounds over the long run.

Saving calories and money

A great way to save calories is to eat more volume. Penn State University professor Barbara Rolls, PhD, calls it *volumetrics,* or consuming higher volume foods for less calories. If you're adding high-fiber, high-water-content foods to your diet, like fruits and veggies, as well as broth-based soups and hot whole-grain cereal, chances are, you're filling up on fewer calories, as well as saving money over the long run. If you think about long-term healthcare costs of managing heart disease or type-2 diabetes — two diseases where the risk goes up with poor eating habits — it makes sense to choose healthful foods to save big bucks later (as well as extend the quality of your life). You may think you're saving money at the cheap fast food restaurants now, but you may be paying the healthcare price later!

You can eat 2 cups of grapes or ½ cup of raisins for the same calories. Which would satisfy you more? The grapes, of course.

Nature has a way of helping out our natural appetites — as well as fending off disease — because the most satiating, water-filled foods are also high in fiber and plant-based nutrients.

The following fruits and vegetables contain 90 percent or higher water:

Broccoli	Eggplant	Sweet peppers
Cabbage	Grapefruit	Tomatoes
Cantaloupe	Spinach	Watermelon
Cauliflower	Strawberries	Zucchini

So, it behooves you to get at least 2 cups of fruit and 2 to 3 cups of vegetables every day!

Part V
The Part of Tens

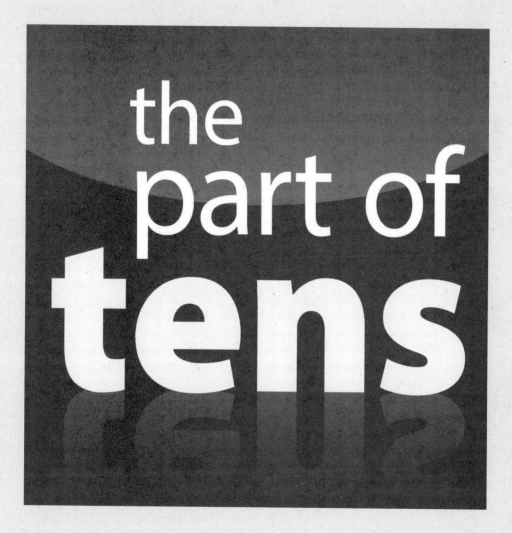

Debunk ten common weight loss myths in a free article at www.dummies.com/extras/totalbodydiet.

In this part . . .

- ✔ Get ten tips on sticking to the Total Body Diet for life.
- ✔ Discover ten tech tools to help you track what you eat, how you sleep, and more.
- ✔ Find ten ways to stay active for total body health.
- ✔ Find ten tips for keeping the weight off after you've lost it.

Chapter 15

Ten Tips for Sticking to the Total Body Diet for Life

*W*ho doesn't need inspiration while on the road to total body health and wellness? They key is following a path that's in sync with your lifestyle at every life stage. Tastes change, hormones fluctuate, and nutritional needs shift as life's landscape expands into new territory. Recalibrating your Total Body Diet plan with the changing tides will help you maintain realistic expectations regardless of your stage in life. In this chapter, I give you ten tips for sticking to the Total Body Diet for years to come.

Taking It One Day at a Time

You really only have this moment. Yesterday is in the past, and tomorrow is still yet to unfold, but today is yours for the taking. The sooner you find joy in the here and now, the better. According to *Present Perfect*, by Pavel Somov, PhD, finding compassion and self-acceptance is a gift you give yourself every day — like a treasure you open on your birthday. Think of the joy that moment brings!

When you feel overwhelmed by the day or disheartened because your eating wasn't in tip-top shape, take a moment and do the following:

> ✔ **Breathe in and out.** In the practice of meditation, breathing is a way to calm the central nervous system, refocus your attention, and find gratitude in the moment. *Meditation For Dummies*, 3rd Edition,

by Stephan Bodian (John Wiley & Sons, Inc.), has a variety of breathing exercises, including a CD for guided meditation. Here's a simple one you can try: Breathe in through the nose for a count of four, and then exhale through the nose for a count of four. Repeat for a few minutes.

- ✔ **Journal your feelings.** Journaling is an effective way of grounding yourself, moving on with your behavior change, and re-evaluating your goals. It helps you focus on this moment, this day. Journaling can help you stick to your Total Body Diet plan by identifying your missteps, addressing what happened, and planning to respond differently in the future.

- ✔ **Take tea time.** A cup of tea soothes the soul. Whether it's hot or cold, sipping tea gives you a reprieve from the hassles of your day. Plus, green tea is packed with antioxidant compounds, primarily one called epigallocatechin gallate (EGCG), which is believed to help defend the body's cells against cancer.

Relishing the Small Successes

Although bigger seems better in today's world, it's really the small stuff that matters. Ordering grilled chicken instead of fried, taking a ten-minute walk on your lunch break, tossing an apple in your work bag for a snack — all these small steps add up. And it's not just about the calories you're saving and burning; the action you take leads to a chain reaction of small successes that lead to healthy habits in the long run.

Relishing small successes requires being aware of the tiny seeds you're sowing every day. Take five-minutes at the end of every day to jot down everything you did that day that contributed to your healthy eating and living goals. Small things like bringing your own lunch to work (and avoiding eating out) or walking to/from work or choosing fruit as a snack over candy add up to big results.

Visualizing Your Goal

Your mind's eye is such a powerful player in making your dreams and goals come true. Ralph Waldo Emerson said it simply: "When there is no vision, people perish." Your Total Body Diet goals are unique to you. Whether your goal is to lose weight, fend off disease, or cook healthier meals for your family, putting a picture to your goal helps.

Visualize what's on your plate — either your literal food plate or your figurative life plate. If you could have the plate of your dreams, what would be on it? It doesn't have to be food necessarily, but for the purposes of the Total Body Diet, it should take into account mental and physical health. Maybe it's a fulfilling career, more energy, a sense of happiness, or the drive to declutter your kitchen to make room for cooking healthier meals? Draw a large circle on a piece of paper to represent your plate. Then write or draw your desired goal(s) on that plate.

Here's another quick visualization exercise:

1. **Get into a comfortable position in a quiet place.**

2. **Clear your mind of the chatter of extra thoughts.**

3. **Imagine achieving (or having) your desired goal.**

4. **Think about how you'll feel when you've attained your goal.**

   This step is a key component of visualization!

When you have *felt* what it's like to reach your goals, repeat this exercise over and over again.

Eating Healthful Food First

It's hard to get away from manufactured food products because they're easy to find and typically inexpensive. According to the Food Marketing Institute, the average number of items carried in a supermarket is 43,844 — and you can bet that many of those items are manufactured food products. That's not to say that manufactured foods are all unhealthy, but minimally processed foods are better! What do I mean by minimally processed? Think vegetables, fruits, whole grains, legumes, lean sources of protein, and lowfat or fat-free dairy products, such as milk, cheese, and yogurt. If you eat healthful foods first, you won't have a lot of room in your stomach for more processed food products.

This tip is simple to say but hard to do. So how can you make this a habit when you're bombarded with processed foods in just about every supermarket? Here are some strategies for making it through the grocery store with a cart full of healthful foods:

- ✔ **Stick to your grocery list.** Planning creates purpose (and helps overcome impulse shopping).

- ✔ **Don't go to the grocery store hungry.** If you're hankering for something, everything looks good!

- ✔ **Read food labels.** Make sure to read those labels *before* you put those items in your cart (not after you bring them home).

- ✔ **Don't fall for sales.** Just because you can get brownies or soda or chips on sale doesn't mean that's a healthy bargain!

Bouncing Back from a Bump in the Road

Bumps are part of every journey, including the Total Body Diet one. The problem comes in when a bump — a night out where overeating ensues, indulging in cookies at work, or stopping for fast food because you didn't plan ahead — throws you off track.

How do you keep yourself from spiraling out of control when things don't go the way you hoped? First, forgive yourself — treat yourself with the same kindness you would show your best friend. Second, remember that the practice of healthy eating is just that: a continual *practice* that isn't perfect. The sooner you get back on the journey of healthy eating, the sooner you'll feel better.

No food is off limits unless it's a *trigger* (a food that sets off overindulgent behavior). If you struggle with this concept, talk to a registered dietitian and/or clinical psychologist who specializes in disordered eating.

Being Open to New Foods

The Total Body Diet is not a rigid food plan. In fact, it's just the opposite — it encourages you to eat an array of healthy foods from vegetables, fruits, grains, proteins, and dairy products, plus healthful fats. To get enough variety in your diet, you may have to try new foods from each of these groups.

If you've never had kiwi or papaya or mandarin oranges, break out of your fruit rut and go for it! If artichoke hearts, broccoli rabe, and baby kale aren't part of your normal routine, give them a try!

If you're a meat eater, try some plant-based proteins like *tofu* (soybean curd), *edamame* (whole soybeans), and *quinoa* (an ancient grain). You may not even miss the meat — and you'll have some good protein alternatives that are lower in saturated fat and jam-packed with plant nutrients.

If you're a dairy fan, why not try *kefir,* a cultured milk product? Not only will you get *probiotics* (friendly bacteria that promote good digestive health), but you'll get a good amount of protein and calcium, too.

Before you know it, as your incorporate new, healthy foods, you'll start to crave these foods that you wouldn't have dreamed of eating before — and you'll find it easier to stick to the Total Body Diet.

Making Sure Your Hormones Don't Rule Your Life

Hormones, especially the sex hormones, get a bad rap for a lot in life — and for good reason. From the moment puberty strikes, it's easy to blame weight gain and cravings on the surge of *estrogen* (the primary sex hormone in females) and *testosterone* (the primary sex hormone in males). Acne, voice changes, and hair growth on armpits and legs sneak up on pubescent adolescents. For women, during pregnancy and afterward into menopause, hormones are key players in mood and behavior.

The more aware you are of how your hormonal changes affect you, the better. For example, if you know that you crave sweets at a certain time of the month, prepare for it — allow yourself a chocolate treat or pastry from your favorite bakery and then be done.

Hormones like *cortisol,* which your adrenal glands release when your stress levels flair up, may affect your eating behaviors, mood, and weight. A study in the journal *European Eating Disorders Review* found increased cortisol levels to be linked to *stress eating* (consuming food or beverages when you aren't necessarily hungry, but as a reaction to what's happening in your life). The researchers found that women over 45 years old with more chronic stress and higher cortisol levels ate fewer vegetables, consumed more food at a buffet, and had more comfort food cravings — all leading to eating more calories and weight gain.

How can you fend off cravings and weight gain, whether they're caused by sex hormones or stress hormones? Eat balanced meals, with no skipping or skimping. Try to include a healthy protein and fat source with every meal and snack. For example, for breakfast have a piece of whole-grain toast with nut butter and a piece of fruit; for lunch, try a wrap with avocado, lettuce, tomato, and a lean protein, such as tuna.

Physical activity is a natural hormone regulator. Moving your body not only improves your mood, but also regulates eating, suppresses cravings, and helps keep weight in check, which in turn helps regulate insulin levels and staves off type-2 diabetes.

Understanding Your Aging Body

Aging is a normal part of life: As soon as you're born, your cells begin to age. The cells you have at birth are not the same ones you have as an adult. According to the National Institute on Aging (NIA), genetics plays a huge role in how we age. Numerous genes are implicated in the normal aging process.

The good news is that older adults are healthier today than ever before, but the risk of diseases and other conditions increases as you get older. Although the process of aging is still not fully clear, one thing is: Your genes, environment, and lifestyle play a big role in how you age. But you can affect change in these areas. What you eat can affect change in your genetic code!

A relatively new area of study called *nutritional genomics* is the study of diet-genome interactions as they relate to chronic disease. It's personalized nutrition at its best!

To keep your cells healthy longer, eat antioxidant-rich foods. Antioxidants (vitamins A, C, E, selenium, and carotenoids) defend cells against the oxidative damage of scavengers called *free radicals*.

Which foods are rich in antioxidants? Colorful fruits, vegetables, nuts, seeds, and eggs. (Egg yolks are high in lutein and zeaxanthin, two carotenoids that deposit in the retina of the eye and help fend off age-related macular degeneration!)

Plant chemicals like resveratrol in the skin of grapes have been shown to be beneficial in fending off vascular inflammation, decreasing the rate of cardiovascular aging. Through a complex process, resveratrol activates cardiac and vascular cellular antioxidant enzymes, which helps lessen damage from free radicals, protecting the heart muscle cells from aging.

Before you go out and drink copious amounts of red wine, remember that you can get too much of a good thing. If you're a woman, aim for one 5-ounce glass of wine a day; if you're a man, two 5-ounce glasses is your max. Too much vino can *increase* your risk for heart disease.

Keep your cell hydrated with water. Aim to drink half your body weight in ounces every day (for example, if you weigh 200 pounds, you should try to get 100 ounces of water a day).

Get physical activity daily — the more you move, the less function you'll lose in your muscles, joints, and ligaments. And you retain your flexibility, too!

Eating Well for Baby and You

Pregnancy is an amazing time in the life of a woman. With your whole body changing and transforming comes new nutritional opportunities and challenges. For many women, this may be the first time health has become a big consideration — having a baby growing inside you is life changing (literally!).

Eating well is vital during pregnancy. Here are some ways to ensure you get adequate nutrition during pregnancy:

✔ **Eat enough calories, but don't go overboard.** Factor in an extra 340 calories per day during your second trimester and an extra 452 calories per day during your third trimester. That's not a lot. Here are some options that fall in that calorie range:

  • A medium piece of fruit with a tablespoon of nut butter

  • An English muffin with a slice of cheese

  • 1 cup of plain nonfat or lowfat yogurt with 1 cup of berries and ¼ cup of chopped walnuts

✔ **Get a variety of healthy foods from all the food groups.** Planning balanced meals and snacks is important when you're pregnant. Get colorful vegetables, fruits, whole grains, lean proteins (from plant and animal sources), as well as lowfat dairy products every day.

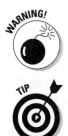

Watch out for fish — steer clear of the large fish: shark, tilefish, king mackerel, and swordfish. Plus, due to its mercury content, limit white albacore tuna to 6 ounces per week.

To get a daily meal plan for pregnancy from the USDA, check out `www.choosemyplate.gov/supertracker-tools/daily-food-plans/moms.html`.

✔ **Get regular, moderate physical activity.** During pregnancy, exercise helps keep blood pressure, blood sugar, and weight gain in a healthy range. Physical activity also keeps muscles and ligaments limber to prepare you for a smooth labor and delivery! Although, pregnancy is not the time to start a rigorous workout routine, getting activity is important. According to the Academy of Nutrition and Dietetics, pregnant women should aim for at least 150 minutes per week of moderate-intensity aerobic activity spread throughout the week. Walking, prenatal yoga, and Pilates all work well.

Saying No When You Need To

Social connection is a healthy part of life, bringing happiness and fostering well-being. So, it makes sense that the Total Body Diet approach advocates a healthy social life. However, if your family, friends, or co-workers are causing you to overeat (or drink too much alcohol) or miss your workouts, it's time to reevaluate. In my counseling practice, I often tell my clients that it's okay to say no to social invitations. I don't want you to be holed up in your home alone, but I do want you to be discerning with your time.

Here some ways to know when it's time to say no:

- ✔ You've gone out two nights in a row, and the third invitation is there.
- ✔ You haven't been able to work out for three consecutive days due to social events.
- ✔ You haven't been able to get to the grocery store all week and plan healthy meals.
- ✔ You're giving into cravings more because you're eating on the run.

If you're declining too many social events or isolating yourself frequently, that's not healthy, either. Finding the right balance between social and alone time is important for your self-esteem and overall well-being. Just knowing you have a choice is empowering!

How about making your healthy lifestyle a part of your social life? Meet a friend for a brisk walk or join an exercise class together. Get together with friends for a cup of tea and challenge each other with a goal-planning session; then meet regularly to keep each other in check (and talk about life!). Go for an after-work run with your buddies instead of meeting for drinks. The Total Body Diet plan works best when it's part of your life!

Chapter 16

Ten Tech Tools for the Total Body Diet

*M*obile devices are a big part of today's fast-paced lifestyle. Ninety percent of American adults own a cellphone, and 64 percent own *smartphones* (mobile phones that can access the Internet with a swipe of a finger). It's now possible to be tapped into the virtual world 24/7, and a recent report by Pew Research Center reveals that people who use smartphones experience positive feelings of productivity and happiness (which is a boost for your total body wellness!). Six out of ten smartphone users use their devices to get information about health conditions.

According to the upcoming book *Bits and Bites: A Guide to Digitally Tracking Your Food, Fitness, and Health* (Eat Right Press), there are tens of thousands of health and fitness mobile apps available, and dozens of wearable devices, too. Mobile tools can help you meet your total body wellness goals by keeping track of

✔ **Daily food intake:** You can track calories and nutrients consumed. Some apps provide nutrition information for restaurant, grocery store, and brand-name foods, as well as connect you with a registered dietitian nutritionist (RDN) to provide feedback on your food choices.

✔ **Fitness levels:** You can track steps and calories burned and even get voice coaching during activities.

✔ **Hydration status:** You can keep tabs on how much water you drink.

> ✔ **Sleep patterns:** Some apps measure circadian rhythms and sleep cycles, which is important because good-quality sleep is linked with preventing chronic diseases.
>
> ✔ **Social support:** Apps can create challenges for friends and family to exercise more and improve food choices.

This chapter highlights some helpful tech tools for total body wellness. This is, by no means, a complete list — new ones are coming out every day! I home in on those with tracking mechanisms that facilitate healthier food choices, meal planning, grocery shopping, physical activity, as well as sleep and mindfulness. These tools are great to use as support and communication for working with an RDN or other healthcare professional.

SuperTracker

SuperTracker (www.supertracker.usda.gov) is the United States Department of Agriculture (USDA) interactive website that helps you plan, analyze, and track your diet and physical activity. It offers accountability through journaling and virtual coaching. You can set personalized goals, and find out what and how much you're eating by tracking foods, physical activities, and weight. You can register on the site for free, and save your personal records so you can come back and access it any time.

This online diet and physical activity tracking website is offered as one of the interactive tools on the MyPlate website (www.choosemyplate.gov), which offers professional and consumer nutrition education. SuperTracker is a fun, eye-catching, broad-based way for folks of all ages to make lifestyle changes to reduce the risk of chronic disease and maintain or achieve a healthy weight. With a variety of features to support personal nutrition and physical activity goals, this website offers

> ✔ Personalized recommendations for what and how much to consume, as well as type and amount of physical activity
>
> ✔ Access to a database of more than 8,000 foods
>
> ✔ Input and analysis of your own recipes
>
> ✔ Tracking of your body weight over time
>
> ✔ Tips and sharing with family and friends via social media
>
> ✔ Journaling personal progress and behavior changes
>
> ✔ Progress reports ranging from simple meal summaries to complex analyses of food groups and nutrient intake over time

MyDietitian

Designed for smartphones, MyDietitian (`www.mydietitian.com`) educates users on the nutritional aspects of their diet through working closely with a registered dietitian nutritionist (RDN). Through food photos and personal accounts, users record on this mobile app (available for download on Apple and Android devices) what they eat and drink, as well as their physical activity, which is passed along within a 24-hour timeline to their assigned RDN for feedback.

MyDietitian establishes a professional relationship with an RDN to offer accountability for what you eat and drink, as well as your level of physical activity. To get results, users are encouraged to log in to the website for their progress reports to view their personal graphs and ratings. Plus, RDNs daily responses can come in the form of videos, emails, or written messages through the app.

This mobile food and fitness tracker allows for real-time tracking with downloadable images of meals and snacks, which creates a connection between the mind and body in every food choice. This tool will become a powerful player for mindful eating, wherever you are!

The app itself is free, but there is a fee associated with the online membership.

Lose It!

Based on the principles of calorie tracking and peer support, Lose It! (`www.loseit.com`; Apple, Android, Kindle, Nook) is a multifaceted system for tracking, connecting, and staying motivated. It allows you to track what you're eating and drinking simply by scanning a bar code, as well as fitness support by connecting with mobile fitness trackers. It offers friend support, but not professional support from an RDN (although you can take the initiative to invite an RDN you're working with to view your logs and send feedback via email).

There are two plans: basic and premium. The basic plan, which is free, allows you to

- ✔ Track your weight.
- ✔ Scan bar codes of food products.
- ✔ Connect with family and friends.
- ✔ Join public groups and challenges.
- ✔ Receive a MyPlate report.

The premium plan, which costs $39.99 per year, allows you to do everything the basic plan allows, plus the following:

- ✔ Monitor body weight, fat, and hydration levels with a Bluetooth scale (for an extra one-time fee of $69.99).
- ✔ Monitor sleep.
- ✔ Track steps and calories burned during exercise.
- ✔ Connect with popular mobile fitness devices (for example, NikeFuel, FitBit One, and JawBone Up).
- ✔ Participate in public and private fitness challenges.

Emeals

As the name implies, Emeals (www.emeals.com; Apple, Android) is a mobile meal planning system designed to assist you in your weekly meal planning with recipes and master shopping lists. The meal plans run the gamut and include Diabetic, Heart Healthy, Low-Calorie, Mediterranean, and more. There are also grocery store–based plans to highlight sale items for that week, as well as family-friendly and quick meal ideas.

It's a simple, highly accessible way to plan meals, but keep in mind that it doesn't take the place of working directly with an RDN. Emeals is a practical way to get weekly meal planning solutions and save time and money. Not only are these healthy, balanced meals, but they offer a wide array of meal plans to fit into your lifestyle and health needs.

Here's how Emeals works, according to the website: You pick your meals, get the recipes correlated to your chosen meal plan, get a detailed shopping list (with sale items if you choose the store-based plan), and prepare the meals.

It costs $69 for one year, $59 for six months, or $39 for three months. You can try it out for free for 14 days, too.

Lark

A virtual personal coach, Lark is a mobile app (Apple, Android) that tracks your activity, eating, and sleep data from sensors in your smartphone. The purpose of the app is to drive you to make healthy lifestyle changes (or continue to do so!) by creating the feeling of a true coach on the other side of your mobile device. It has an upbeat, positive voice encouraging you to get more sleep or make healthier food choices. You can compare how you're doing with other Lark community members, too!

If you have your mobile device with you, this app offers two-way motivation with automated conversations and text messages. It adapts to your schedule with a unique quality to show you how to manage travel and jet lag, offers tips to get more sleep, and sets up charts and graphs of your activity and sleep patterns. You can tell this app what you're eating — and it will respond with instant feedback.

It may seem like a lark to have artificial intelligence leading the way in the mobile health app arena, but it has shown to be beneficial for motivation and accountability in today's fast-paced world. Lark follows you where you go and texts and responds to your voice with motivational charts and creative solutions to eating and fitness dilemmas. It can be a great adjunct therapy in between visiting with an RDN or other healthcare team member. There is a support community on social media, too — members use the hashtag #larkgoals.

MyFitnessPal

This free website and app (www.myfitnesspal.com; Apple, Android) is all about tracking what you eat to help you lose weight. With more than 5 million foods in its database, MyFitnessPal offers you a simple and easy way to be mindful of what you're putting in your mouth every day. You set your own personal weight loss goals and keep track of your food and beverage intake in order to stay within your nutrition and calorie goals for the day.

Tracking what you eat and drink is ideal, and MyFitnessPal allows you do just that. It creates mindfulness and can help keep you from overeating (and listening to hunger and fullness), if you know that you're going to write it down. Plus, tuning into your physical activity and making sure it happens is essential to weight management. Although there is an online forum for support, this weight loss tool may be more beneficial if paired with an RDN to offer professional feedback and nutrition solutions. (You can eat whatever you want within your goal calorie range, but that doesn't mean it's a healthy, balanced approach to help prevent chronic diseases down the road!)

Whether you are logging your food and activity on your home computer or want to do it on the go with your mobile device, MyFitnessPal allows you the opportunity to see the nutritional value of what was on your plate, according to the portion that was consumed. It has a recall feature, which remembers your favorite foods, too — making it easy to log your typical breakfast or lunch without taking a lot of time or effort. This may promote lack of variety, though, so watch out for that!

Sleep Genius

Having trouble falling or staying asleep? Sleep Genius may be the app for you — it offers a scientific approach to creating a restful sleep environment and healthy bedtime behaviors (also called *sleep hygiene*), and pinpoints your perfect bedtime. The sleep technology in this app (available for Apple and Android devices) uses elements to engage the brain's sleep centers by combining expertise from neuroscientists, as well as sleep and music experts.

Because sleep health is such a vital part of your overall total body wellness, Sleep Genius is an important tool to help you get much needed rest. Lack of sleep has been linked to the development and management of chronic diseases, according to the Centers for Disease Control and Prevention. Sleep Genius also homes in on the power of naps and encourages brief periods of shuteye throughout the day with a Power Nap feature that offers sleep-inducing music to relax you and an alarm to gradually wake you up.

Through a specialized sleep sound system, which includes special beats, brain-relaxing music, as well *pink noise* (sounds that block out distracting noises), Sleep Genius is set up to encourage the brain to fall asleep faster, deeper, and longer. In addition, it targets the right bedtime for you — this sleep technology trains you (and your brain) to go to bed within 15 minutes of your targeted bedtime. Plus, a soothing alarm is embedded into the system, which allows you to awaken slowly without harsh, startling noise. You also get sleep reports to assess your sleep quality to be able to make improvements accordingly.

The app is $4.99 plus add-ons for Sleep Genius Audio Programs.

Before I Eat, Moment in the Zone

Getting into the zone before eating can be a powerful player in making healthy food choices — and not overeating. This app with a long name (available for $0.99 for Apple devices) is geared toward managing food cravings and stopping urges in their tracks, as they occur. Through a collection of audio sessions and other resources, Before I Eat, Moment in the Zone, offers you mindful eating strategies.

The beauty of this app is that it allows you space to stop, breathe, and think before eating. It teaches you ways to surf urges beyond the traditional behavior therapy techniques with inspirational quotes, guided audio sessions, and countdown timers for quick focus. Plus, it offers tips for countering emotional eating triggers. You can track your progress on the app, and it even offers rewards for success, such as money toward a vacation fund or 15 minutes of guilt-free TV (you can also create your own rewards). The only downside is some of the sessions are as long as nine minutes, which can be a bit lengthy.

To start off, there's a tutorial teaching you how to navigate the app. You can create your own plan. This app introduces a concept called HALT-B, which stands for the following and offers the simple solutions:

Hungry? Think mindfully.

Angry/Anxious? Try to relax.

Lonely/Sad? Food is not comfort.

Tired? Get some rest.

Bored? Busy yourself.

With an option to journal, set goals, and take notes, this app is designed to work with eating urges. It offers guidance and progress rating with a star system (on a scale of one to five stars).

HAPIfork

Want to eat more mindfully and slowly? HAPIfork may be for you. HAPIfork (www.hapi.com; Apple, Android) is an actual fork with an electronic device in it that counts the number of bites that goes from your plate to your mouth. If you're having more than one bite every 10 seconds, a light indicator goes on to help you realize that you need to slow down your eating. Plus, you can link this tool to your computer and track the speed at which you're eating or time between fork servings, as well as overall eating for the day.

If you're craving mindful eating, this is the mobile device for you. In a world where mindless eating abounds, HAPIfork can offer you a solution to slowing down your eating. There's a coaching program that goes along with HAPIfork, in which you can connect with professionals — an RDN would be a great adjunct here — to motivate you along your path to mindful, healthier eating and living.

There are a couple of drawbacks: You have to have the fork with you when you eat, so don't forget it at home when you go to work or school or a lunch date. Plus, if you aren't not eating foods that require a fork, you can't use it!

The app allows for accountability in real time, while you're eating. You can sync it up to a whole community on www.hapi.com to see your dashboard, which can track your daily eating and fitness goals, participate in challenges, and share with friends.

HAPIfork can tell you:

- ✔ How long it took you to eat your meal
- ✔ The amount of fork servings taken per minute
- ✔ The time between fork servings

You can see your fork stats on the www.hapi.com dashboard, because it's all uploaded via USB or Bluetooth from the fork.

The HAPIfork isn't cheap — it costs $79 with a case and micro-USB cable for charging and data upload.

Meallogger

Meallogger is an app (Apple, Android) where you journal with food photos and connect with your friends to exchange thoughts, ideas, and motivation. You can record eating and physical activity goals, share links, and build awareness and accountability for your eating choices.

The app creates real-time accountability and mindful eating. Images are such a powerful tool, and Meallogger makes use of the fun nature of snapping food photos, while at the same time managing your waistline and food choices — but tracking the food and beverage amounts is important. Plus, it may help reduce mindless snacking if you're snapping photos every time you eat or drink! It's all about community support, too — Meallogger can connect you with a professional, too. For example, you can connect with an RDN while on the go. Meallogger makes food journaling simple because there's no real writing involved — just snapping photos and recording the contents. Also, it encompasses the whole body with the fitness and sleep components.

You can track calories, carbohydrates, and protein for each meal, if you input portion sizes. The basic program (which is free) affords you a connection to friends; for a premium, you can connect with professionals, whether RDNs, health coaches, or personal trainers. There is a professional version called MealloggerPRO, which allows RDNs to connect directly to their clients for support, too.

Chapter 17

Ten Ways to Stay Active

There's no doubt that a body in motion is healthier and happier. How much activity should you get? The Physical Activity Guidelines for Americans recommend that adults get at least 150 minutes of moderate-intensity aerobic activity (such as brisk walking) or 75 minutes of vigorous-intensity aerobic activity (such as jogging) per week. Strength training that uses all large muscle groups — arms, legs, hips, back, abdomen, chest — is encouraged at least twice a week.

Anything that gets your body moving counts and can offer health benefits!

An active lifestyle is good for your total body wellness and fosters a mind–body connection. Activity can help you focus, think more clearly, and hone your creativity. By moving your body regularly, you not only get cardiovascular benefits, but your blood sugar, blood pressure, and body weight will most likely stay in a healthy range.

Check with your healthcare provider before starting an exercise regimen — especially if you've been diagnosed with diabetes, heart disease, or osteoarthritis or have symptoms like dizziness, chest pain or pressure, or joint pain. Always begin slowly and gradually move from lower- to higher-intensity workouts.

This chapter fills you in on ten fun ways to get moving. From hitting the pavement to the water to the ice rink to the mat, in any season, weather, or mood, there's an activity for you. The best part: You can mix and match activities to give your body a well-rounded variety of activities to shake off boredom and train different muscles groups for total body fitness from head to toe. Let's get moving!

Running

With a good pair of running shoes, you can hit the ground running anytime, anywhere. That's the best part about this activity — it requires very minimal gear.

Whether you're running on a treadmill, track, or paved road, you're getting a cardiovascular workout. However, the open road is different from a treadmill. Running pros use both for different reasons. Here's how they differ:

- **You get better leg muscle conditioning from road running.** Experts believe it works the soft tissues of the legs more because the road doesn't give as much as the treadmill surface does.

- **You can pace your running better on a road than you can on a treadmill.** Although a treadmill pushes you along, the road allows you to gain a better understanding of your own body's pace. So, as you work up to longer runs, it's best to get out on the open road to get a sense of your body's real running time.

- **You get better weather awareness while running on the road.** You're forced to deal with weather conditions like wind, rain, cold, and heat, which helps you prepare for race day weather conditions (if you're preparing for a road race like a 10K or marathon).

- **You're more in control of the workout conditions with a treadmill.** You can run on a treadmill regardless of how bad the weather is outside.

- **You get a heightened sense of speed and tempo from running on a treadmill than you do on the road.** You can vary your running speed, incline, and tempo more easily. You can also do *interval training* (where you alternate the intensity of exertions from greater to lighter) more easily on a treadmill.

Running shoes can make or break your fitness routine. Get a pair that fits your feet well and supports your running style. Your shoes should fit snug, but not be too tight. It's a good idea to have your gait looked at while trying on shoes to determine which shoes will be the best for you.

Walking

Like running, walking requires very little gear — just a good pair of shoes and proper attire for an outdoor excursion. Whether you're walking on a treadmill, outside, or even at the mall, to get the full benefits of walking, make sure you're walking with purpose.

Different from a slow, Sunday stroll, walking for a cardiovascular benefit and to shed some pounds requires a bit of speed and putting your whole body into it. Think about walking home from a job interview that you just aced. You've got your head held high, shoulders back, and legs moving at a good, speedy pace. You're walking on sunshine, with attitude and confidence. That's walking the total body walk!

 Wear a pedometer to track your steps. Strive for 10,000 steps a day — from the moment you wake up until you go to sleep at night. Add a bit of core strength to your walks by intentionally tightening your abdominal muscles with every step. This strategy can prevent injuries, too.

Swimming

There's something magical about immersing your body in water. Your body feels light as it becomes buoyant. Swimming offers the best of both worlds: You can get a good workout for your heart and major muscle groups, and take it easy on your joints at the same time. Whatever stroke you prefer — freestyle, butterfly, backstroke, breast stroke — you'll get a great workout!

Here's why swimming is great for your total body:

- ✔ It allows you to control and focus on breathing for relaxation.
- ✔ It builds endurance and stamina.
- ✔ It develops your major muscle groups (which is great for burning calories once out of the water!).
- ✔ It's low impact (which means it's easy on your joints).
- ✔ The water is soothing and meditative, making for a great escape from stress.

Although swimming a great solo activity (as long as a lifeguard is present), doing it with friends can be a great way to have more fun. Join a local swimming club, if none of your friends are into swimming.

Here are some swimming tips to keep in mind:

- ✔ Always warm up beforehand by walking in place or doing some light squats and cool down afterward with a short walk in or out of the water to avoid injury and reduce muscle tension.
- ✔ Take the time to get your stroke techniques down so that you have good swimming form and can reap the maximum benefits. Use a coach to help you learn the proper technique.

Bike Riding

In Europe, bicycle riding is as common as driving. From the cities to the countryside, riding a bicycle is a mode of transportation for the young and old alike. Cycling is a great form of exercise and has become a competitive sport around the globe.

Even if you learned to ride a bike when you were a kid, before you hop on a bike for exercise, keep in mind a few important points:

- ✔ **Always wear a properly fitting helmet when biking to ensure safety.** Go to a local bike shop for help finding a helmet that fits.

- ✔ **Sit up as straight as you can when cycling.** Hunching your shoulders or tucking your chin when you bike will cause muscle soreness and fatigue.

- ✔ **If there's a designated bike lane or path, use it.** That's why it's there.

- ✔ **Keep a safe distance between you and other bikers.**

- ✔ **Make sure your bike fits your body.** The handlebar width should equal your shoulder width for adequate breathing and handling of the bicycle.

- ✔ **Bring a water bottle and a healthy snack (for example, a small banana plus a handful of nuts, or a peanut butter and jelly sandwich) to fuel your body well, especially if you're cycling longer than an hour.**

Yoga

Dating back thousands of years, yoga is spiritual discipline that teaches meditation, postures, and breathing techniques. It has been shown to decrease stress and depression, help minimize pain from diseases like cancer, and create positive behavior change. The premise of yoga is to create an inner awareness through self-observation without judgment. Through the premise of compassionately accepting yourself, yoga allows change to happen in your life by tapping into your inner wisdom or voice.

Among other health benefits, yoga may have the capacity to stop aging in your brain. A recent study in *Frontiers in Human Neuroscience* examined the gray matter in the brain of longtime *yogis* (people who practice yoga) with a control group of people who didn't practice yoga. The study showed that the control group had significantly higher age-related decline in gray matter in their brains, whereas people who practice yoga did not show the same level of gray matter decline. The researchers surmised that yogis' brains are tuned into the parasympathetic-driven mode — the part of your nervous system that restores your body to a calm state, protecting the brain from aging. By getting quiet with yourself and just being, you can affect positive healthy changes in your mind and body.

You don't have to be an experienced yogi to enjoy the practice of yoga. All different ages, fitness levels, and personality types do yoga. When choosing a type of yoga that's right for you, think about *your* fitness level, what you want out of it (for example, to build strength and muscle tone or to explore the mind-body connection), and your overall health (do you have any injuries or physical limitations?). The best bet is to start with a gentle type and progress to harder or more challenging types of yoga.

Table 17-1 is a quick guide to some types of yoga and what they offer.

Table 17-1		Types of Yoga
Type of Yoga	*Level*	*What It Is*
Hatha	Gentle	Good for beginners. Focuses on the breathing as the yoga practice, more than the poses.
Iyengar	Gentle	Slow-paced and good for beginners. You use blocks, belts, and pillow-like bolsters.
Kripalu	Gentle	Begin with slow movements and progress to a deeper mind-body awareness.
Viniyoga	Gentle	Focus on how your breath moves through your body. It's less about getting the pose perfect and more about gaining flexibility and restoring function. Good for beginners.
Sivananda	Gentle	Thirteen poses. Lie down in between the poses. Good for all physical ability levels.
Kundalini	Gentle	The most meditative type yoga. Allows for spiritual awareness through meditation, breathing, and chanting, along with gentle poses.
Ashtanga	Challenging	Nonstop poses and special breathing techniques.
Bikram	Challenging	Series of 26 poses in a hot room (over 100 degrees).
Power	Challenging	The most athletic type. Flow from one pose to another to build upper-body strength, flexibility, and balance.

Ever wonder how to do a downward dog or warrior or child's pose? Check out the ten yoga poses at `http://fit.webmd.com/teen/move/slideshow/slideshow-yoga-for-energy`. These poses can be energizing and restorative, and generate a mind–body connection instantly.

Yoga teaches gratitude for your life and world. Every yoga class ends with your hands in the prayer position over your heart and the word *namaste* (*nah*-ma-stay), which connects the divine spirit in you with everyone and thing around you. Namaste to you!

For more on yoga, check out *Yoga For Dummies,* 3rd Edition, by Larry Payne, PhD, and Georg Feuerstein, PhD (Wiley).

Pilates

Created by Joseph Pilates (puh-*lah*-teez) in the early 1900s, this method of exercise is a series of mat-work moves typically done kneeling, lying, or sitting to put less strain on the heart and lungs. Pilates offers strength-training, flexibility, and core work through balance and control of the body, which transcends the mat into other areas of your life.

Every age group can participate in Pilates. Know your own fitness level and what you want to gain from it. Pilates emphasizes correct form as opposed to going for the muscle burn. It's about engaging your whole body and concentrating on individual moves physically and mentally. There are different variations of every movement that challenge you to master one and then move to a more difficult one. Pilates focuses on toning muscles with bands, springs, and even better, your own body weight.

To get the most out of your time on the mat, look for a good Pilates teacher who is well trained and has received certification through a reputable organization like the Pilates Method Alliance (www.pilatesmethodalliance.org).

For a whole book dedicated to Pilates, check out *Pilates For Dummies,* by Ellie Herman (Wiley).

Cross-Training

Working different muscle groups with cross-training is ideal. Cross-training facilities are springing up all over the country, helping people to increase their capability and capacity over a broader range of movements and activities. Whether you're an avid cyclist crossing over into running or a runner crossing into swimming, cross-training inherently allows you to train different body parts and build endurance at any fitness level.

The key to good cross-training is to focus on activities that use different body parts and rotate these activities throughout the week or month. To reduce injury, doing this type of activity will help foster strength, flexibility, and endurance in your total body, maximizing athletic performance, cardiovascular health, and weight management over the long term. If you're interested in finding a cross-training program near you, try CrossFit at www.crossfit.com.

Skating

Whether on ice, pavement, or in a roller rink, skating is a great activity for cardiovascular health and to build up your large leg muscles. Skating burns a lot of calories — which makes it a great weight loss and maintenance activity. All types of skating are low-impact, which means it's a joint-friendly workout.

There are risk associated with all types of skating. Learning how to fall is key, especially in ice skating, where you probably aren't wearing a helmet. People who inline skate typically wear plenty of safety gear, like knee pads, elbow pads, wrist pads, and helmets.

All types of skating offer a total body workout because they combine fun and fitness.

Climbing

In recent years, climbing has become very popular. Whether you climb rocks outdoors, or go to an indoor climbing gym and climb on walls, this activity is great for the arms and legs. Climbing is a great way to condition your abdominal, arm, and leg muscles. It's also great for fostering a mind–body connection because it requires a solo force of will to catapult your body up a steep rock, mountain, or manmade edifice.

Some climbing feats are thousands of feet up, making them not only challenging, but death defying. But you don't have to be a daredevil to climb — you can easily recreationally climb at your local climbing wall.

Interested in competitive climbing? Check out the International Federation of Sport Climbing at www.ifsc-climbing.org.

Stretching

One of the most important exercises you can do is stretching — it goes hand in hand with any activity. After you've warmed up your muscles with running, biking, skating, yoga, Pilates, or rock climbing, stretching comes into play. It soothes, conditions, and strengthens muscle fibers to gear them up for rest, growth, and development.

The primary thing that stretching does is improves flexibility. Why is flexibility so important? Because it does the following:

- ✔ **Allows you to do everyday tasks like tying your shoes, putting clothes high up in your closet, and putting away groceries.** Plus, it makes the harder tasks like throwing a football into the end zone or reaching up to catch a fly ball possible.

- ✔ **Minimizes injury as muscles and joints are better conditioned and have moved through a full range of motion, putting less strain on them.**

- ✔ **Enables good circulation, which allows working muscles to get nutrients and recover more quickly.**

- ✔ **Gives you good posture.** Strong muscles will help keep your posture in top form.

There are numerous stretches for every body part from head to toe. Take a look at the stretching guide at www.stretching-exercises-guide.com for the ways to stretch each body part. Or check out *Stretching For Dummies,* by LaReine Chabut (Wiley), for a whole book dedicated to this important subject.

Chapter 18

Ten Tips for Keeping the Weight Off

. . . .

In This Chapter

▶ Uncovering real-life solutions to weight maintenance

▶ Discovering daily motivational tools to overcome temptations

▶ Balancing food, activity, and daily life

. . . .

*T*he road to weight loss and maintenance is a well-beaten path, with arrows pointing in many different directions promising success, but then dead-ending with unrealistic goals and rigid food rules. The quick-fix, fad-diet path seems promising in the beginning, but then it's too good-to-be-true nature seeps in and the realities of individual taste and preferences take over.

Maintaining a healthy body weight throughout life is a vital part of staying healthy. Two out of three people in the United States are overweight or obese, so finding permanent ways to lose weight and keep it off is a public health imperative. Carrying too much weight around not only is uncomfortable, but also can lead to multiple chronic diseases and conditions, such as type-2 diabetes, heart disease, high blood pressure, stroke, and cancer (especially breast cancer and colon cancer). So, what can you do today to stay on a successful weight-loss path for life?

A ten-year study in the *American Journal of Preventive Medicine* examined the weight-loss route of weight losers in the National Weight Control Registry (NWCR), the largest investigation tracking more than 10,000 individuals of long-term successful weight loss maintenance, who lost more than 30 pounds and kept it off for at least one year. In fact, 87 percent of the 2,886 participants maintained at least 10 percent weight loss five and ten years later. How did they do it? Consistent behavior changes long after the weight came off.

In this chapter, I offer up ten tips to help you effectively keep weight off in a realistic and healthy way.

Keep a Food Diary

It sounds so simple: Write down what you eat and drink every day to create awareness of your consumption patterns and encourage healthful choices. A food diary fosters a sense of accountability — to yourself.

But does writing down what you eat really work? A study in *Psychology and Health* found that food diaries work for weight maintenance. Researchers recruited undergraduate students from the University of Greece to join in three studies, which used food diaries to induce mindfulness and self-compassion. They compared concrete (*how* they're eating) diaries with abstract (*why* they're eating) diaries and found that at a three-month follow-up, the students who continued to keep the concrete diaries performed better at weight maintenance. Also, the researchers surmised that the food diaries may encourage more mindfulness and self-compassion, which potentially promotes weight loss in the long run.

So, what are some quick and simple ways to stick with a food diary day in and day out? Here are some Total Body Diet suggestions:

- ✔ Keep a notebook by your bedside or desk at work to make it easy to jot down meals and snacks.

- ✔ Create a simple food log on your computer or smartphone to simply note what you eat and drink.

- ✔ Use the voice recorder on your smartphone to keep track of your intake and how you feel before and after eating.

- ✔ Take advantage of the myriad food diary apps or websites and record your foods and feelings that way. You can even take photos with some apps, making it even easier!

Plan, Plan, Plan

Planning creates purpose. If you have a plan, you're more likely to stick with it. Mindless eating comes in when there's no structure. Weight gain can occur when the future is unclear, but if you've planned your meals and snacks for the day, there's less chance of overeating and more security in keeping your weight stable. When left up in the air, food choices become knee-jerk reactions, in-the-moment decisions — and that typically doesn't go very well.

If you aren't a natural planner, take stock: Planning can be learned. When you start to plan, it becomes second nature. Start with balancing meals and snacks with healthful foods from the food groups: whole grains, vegetables, fruits, proteins, lowfat dairy products.

Plan to *not* plan at least one day a week. This unplanned day will allow you flexibility and renew your focus for the rest of the week.

Cook the Healthy Way

Unfortunately, cooking does not top the list of priorities for the average American. If you had four extra hours in the day, would you cook more? Not so much, according to the International Food Information Council Foundation's 2015 Food & Nutrition Survey.

The good news is, you need only 20 to 30 minutes to make a tasty and healthy meal! And you don't have to be a trained chef to cook healthy meals. There are so many culinary learning outlets today — from cooking schools to websites to how-to videos, the list of ways to get into the kitchen are endless. Cooking can be fun and a great way to try news foods and bond with family and friends. Experimenting with new herbs and spices, plant-based proteins, a multitude of whole grains, and vegetables and fruits will expand your nutritional repertoire, too. It's liberating to create recipes from scratch or place your personal taste stamp on someone else's recipe!

If you're relying on dining out for nourishing meals, the promising news is that culinary trends reveal a focus in food that is good for both the planet and health. According to the National Restaurant Association 2015 Culinary Forecast, which polled 1,300 chefs nationwide, locally sourced meats and seafood, locally grown produce, natural ingredients, and minimally processed foods top the list of current hot foods trends. Translating these trends to your home kitchen can help you create your own healthy meals, plus help reign in your calorie budget (and financial budget, too)!

Eating at home bodes better for your waistline — as well as cuts salt, saturated fat, and sugar consumption. A recent article published in Public Health Nutrition using data from the National Health & Nutrition Examination Survey looked at nutrition and dining habits of 12,000 American adults. The study findings revealed that regardless of where you dine out — fast food or full-service restaurant — you'll eat at least 200 calories more per day, plus sugar, fat, and sodium intake soars when dining out.

Here are five simple ways to get cooking that don't take a lot of time:

- ✔ Gather a repertoire of three or four recipes that are simple to make and use them throughout the week. Grocery shop for the week with your recipes in mind.

- ✔ Limit your recipes to five ingredients total. Feel free to swap ingredients — such as different fruits, vegetables, proteins, grains, or herbs and spices — to add variety to your meals and snacks.

✔ Cook with family and friends to make it more fun!

✔ Play music while you cook to relax into the process.

✔ Dabble and try new flavors with herbs and spices, vegetables, fruits, nuts, and beans. Enjoy a bounty of good food in your kitchen!

Steer Clear of Temptations

I'm all for allowing yourself small indulgences, but what about foods that cause you to *binge* (excessively indulge to the point that it's hard to stop)? These foods or beverages are often called *triggers* because they set off a period of overindulgence. Usually, these foods and drinks don't have a lot of nutritional value, and your brain and body are craving the *feeling* they give you. (Think sugary beverages, cakes, cookies, candy, or alcohol, as well as salty chips, dips, and fries.)

Set a steer-clear attitude — not a restrictive one:

✔ **Clear your home of tempting foods or beverages.**

✔ **Replace unhealthy foods and beverages with healthier, individually portioned substitutes.** For example, if you like soda, get some mineral water and add lemon or lime. If it's chocolate you're after, buy an individually wrapped dark chocolate square and savor one. If chips are your kryptonite, get an individual bag of baked chips and enjoy with a turkey and avocado wrap for lunch. And instead of dessert after dinner, have a piece of fruit or a bowl of berries to end the meal.

✔ **Share with family and friends.** Sharing creates more from less. If you're dining out and you usually get dessert and wind up overeating, share a dessert with your spouse, friends, or family. Just think: You'll eat less overall and get the feeling of more that comes from sharing!

Establish a Supportive Structure

Surrounding yourself with social support is key when you're trying to lose weight and maintain weight loss. Think about it: Who can help you on your journey to a healthy lifestyle? Your place on the path to health and wellness may be different from your neighbor's or friend's place, but knowing that you're are all here together trying to attain health, happiness, and longevity is a great source of support.

Resiliency in life and with weight maintenance requires reaching out for support, even though it can be hard at times. Try naming at least one person who can help you in each of the following situations:

✔ When you're tempted by food at work

✔ When you want to stop at your favorite fast-food restaurant on the way home from work

✔ When your neighbors invite you to a party where you know there will be a lot of food and alcohol

✔ When you want to blow off your workout

✔ When you're dining out with friends and you're tempted to overeat

Are there people you can reach out to for help talking through the eating challenges that these situations may impose? If so, reach out to them in times of need. If you can't come up with anyone to help you, reach out to your healthcare provider or a registered dietitian nutritionist (RDN) for professional assistance. Visit www.eatright.org to find an RDN in your area.

Check in with Yourself

How you feel about your food choices is just as important as the actual food on your plate. That's why checking in with yourself to see how you feel is so important. At first, you may find it challenging because you'd rather eat waffles than oatmeal, but making a compromise by switching to whole-grain waffles will allow you to feel much more content with your choice.

The Total Body Diet isn't about eliminating your favorite foods — it's about allowing you to stretch your taste buds by making new, healthy choices. You may never even have thought of making vegetable chili with beans instead of meat or replacing a sugary, gourmet coffee drink with a cup of green tea for a soothing, stress-relieving reprieve during your workday.

Ask yourself the following questions throughout the day:

✔ Do I feel satisfied *right now* with my food and beverage choice?

✔ Could I have made this a more mindful experience?

✔ What new health-enhancing food can I try today?

✔ Am I eating with awareness of my choices?

If a day goes by in which you don't check in, just get back on the horse — now. There's no greater time than the present to appreciate the moment. You'll be happy you did!

Savor Good Foods and Flavors

Eating on autopilot doesn't allow for savoring and really *tasting* foods with their amazing bevy of flavors. If you think about it, when you go to a tasting class — whether it's wine, cheese, or chocolate — the flavors on your tongue ignite as you stop and slowly allow the food or beverage to dissipate.

To savor means to taste and enjoy the food or drink completely. The slow, deliberate act of tasting excites the senses and creates an extraordinary experience.

So, how can you more fully savor what you eat and drink? By understanding the concept of *taste-specific satiety* also called *sensory-specific satiety* — the notion that your taste buds are chemical receptors that tire over time. In other words, the first few bites or sips of a drink taste the best on your tongue (and should be savored!). With every bite, a food's taste begins to dull and your tongue is soon in search of another taste sensation. This can be dangerous to your waistline, if you keep seeking flavor and eat until uncomfortably full. Instead, create mindful bites, savor small tastes, and listen to your hunger and fullness.

You can train your taste buds to enjoy less sugar, salt, and fat over time. As you begin eating less salty, sugary, and fatty foods, your palette becomes used to it. When you eat a salty, sugary, or fatty food again, it's a shock to your system. You're training your palette that less is more!

Stay Active Every Day

According to the International Food Information Council Foundation's 2015 Food & Nutrition Survey, if given four more hours every day, 36 percent of respondents would use that time to exercise more! Exercise is one of the top ways to maintain weight throughout a lifetime. You don't have to spend a lot of time working out, either. Activity can come in many forms and in short bursts — ten-minute increments spaced throughout the day can do wonders for your mind, body, and spirit!

Before beginning any new physical activity consult with your healthcare provider. Start small, with light activity, and then progress to the harder stuff. Aim for 150 minutes per week.

Here are some ideas for short-burst, ten-minute activities:

- Ride your bike to and from a corner store.
- Walk your dog around the block.
- Jog to and from the mailbox.
- Hula-hoop to music.
- Dance to your favorite song.
- Hit the mat for push-ups, sit-ups, and/or planks.

Laughter burns calories, too — and it can boost immunity, alleviate stress, and reduce muscle tension in your body. Research in the *International Journal of Obesity* found that 10 to 15 minutes of laughter a day can burn 10 to 40 calories. That adds up over time — to the tune of 2 to 4 pounds of weight loss in a year (when laughter is combined with your regular physical activity)!

Eat Balanced Meals and Snacks

Combining lean sources of protein with high-fiber carbohydrates and healthy fats helps keep blood sugar in check, fends off cravings, and can help to decrease the chance of overeating and weight gain.

One food, meal, or snack does not make or break a healthy diet — it's the balance of food groups over time that counts. According to the Academy of Nutrition and Dietetics' position paper, Total Diet Approach to Healthy Eating, and the 2010 Dietary Guidelines for Americans, the overall pattern of food eaten is the most important focus of healthy eating. The goal of the Total Body Diet is to place less emphasis on foods to avoid and more emphasis on foods to add for health, happiness, and vitality for life.

Think about balancing the *nutrient density* (the quality of the calories you consume) with what you expend with physical activity. Aim to include more foods that will give you greater nutritional bang for the calories. Plus, think about the form of the foods — when a healthy food like grapes are dried in raisin form, you get less for the calories. The greater the volume on your plate, the more satisfied you'll be for the same number of calories!

Nutrient-dense foods to include in your day include: vegetables, fruits, whole grains, fat-free and lowfat dairy products, seafood, lean meats, poultry, eggs, beans and peas, nuts, and seeds.

Allow Small Indulgences

Part of balancing your eating and drinking is allowing some of your favorites — moderately and mindfully. There's nothing wrong with having a cookie, chocolate, or ice cream, but it's how often — and *how much* — you eat that counts. The 2010 Dietary Guidelines for Americans refers to these extra calories that are made of solid fats and added sugars as "empty calories." These foods don't provide a lot of nutrients for the amount of calories they contain, which is why eating these foods sparingly and slowly is important.

Your parents offered sage advice when they told you to eat your vegetables, fruits, proteins, and grains on your plate before reaching for a sweet treat. After you've eaten a day's worth of nutrient-rich foods, indulging in a decadent, calorie-controlled treat is perfectly acceptable.

Here are guidelines for a small indulgence:

- ✔ Eat nutrient-rich foods beforehand.
- ✔ Calorie-control the indulgence (150 to 200 calories is enough).
- ✔ Choose food over liquid indulgences — you'll enjoy it more and chewing food will force you to slow down.
- ✔ Don't forget to write your indulgence on your food diary. Include how you felt before and after eating it.
- ✔ Enjoy the indulgence guilt-free!

Metric Conversion Guide

· ·

*N**ote:* The recipes in this book weren't developed or tested using metric measurements. There may be some variation in quality when converting to metric units.

Common Abbreviations

Abbreviation(s)	What It Stands For
cm	Centimeter
C., c.	Cup
G, g	Gram
kg	Kilogram
L, l	Liter
lb.	Pound
mL, ml	Milliliter
oz.	Ounce
pt.	Pint
t., tsp.	Teaspoon
T., Tb., Tbsp.	Tablespoon

Volume

U.S. Units	Canadian Metric	Australian Metric
¼ teaspoon	1 milliliter	1 milliliter
½ teaspoon	2 milliliters	2 milliliters
1 teaspoon	5 milliliters	5 milliliters
1 tablespoon	15 milliliters	20 milliliters
¼ cup	50 milliliters	60 milliliters
⅓ cup	75 milliliters	80 milliliters
½ cup	125 milliliters	125 milliliters
⅔ cup	150 milliliters	170 milliliters
¾ cup	175 milliliters	190 milliliters
1 cup	250 milliliters	250 milliliters
1 quart	1 liter	1 liter
1½ quarts	1.5 liters	1.5 liters
2 quarts	2 liters	2 liters
2½ quarts	2.5 liters	2.5 liters
3 quarts	3 liters	3 liters
4 quarts (1 gallon)	4 liters	4 liters

Weight

U.S. Units	Canadian Metric	Australian Metric
1 ounce	30 grams	30 grams
2 ounces	55 grams	60 grams
3 ounces	85 grams	90 grams
4 ounces (¼ pound)	115 grams	125 grams
8 ounces (½ pound)	225 grams	225 grams
16 ounces (1 pound)	455 grams	500 grams (½ kilogram)

Length

Inches	Centimeters
0.5	1.5
1	2.5
2	5.0
3	7.5
4	10.0
5	12.5
6	15.0
7	17.5
8	20.5
9	23.0
10	25.5
11	28.0
12	30.5

Temperature (Degrees)

Fahrenheit	Celsius
32	0
212	100
250	120
275	140
300	150
325	160
350	180
375	190
400	200
425	220
450	230
475	240
500	260

Index

N

Notes

Notes

Notes

Notes

Notes

Notes

About the Author

Victoria Shanta Retelny, RDN, LDN, and "The Lifestyle Nutritionist" is a nationally recognized lifestyle nutrition expert, author, and culinary and media consultant. Vicki is the author of *The Essential Guide to Healthy Healing Foods,* an empowering evidence-based exploration into the landscape of food, which encourages readers to evolve their eating for improved health, happiness, and longevity. Vicki has written dozens of nutrition-related articles for national publications, including *The Costco Connection, EatingWell Magazine, Chicago Health Magazine,* MyRecipes.com, *The Chicago Tribune,* and *Today's Dietitian.* Vicki contributes her expertise to media outlets, such as WGN-TV's *Medical Watch,* CBS-TV, and ABC-TV in Chicago.

Vicki runs a private nutrition communications consulting practice in Chicago, in which she counsels clients, as well as offers motivational presentations for companies and conferences. She also partners with food companies as a culinary nutrition and media consultant. She has a passion for translating nutrition science into usable, real-life messages to educate consumers on appreciating healthful ingredients and delicious flavors while creating tasty, nutritious meals at home.

Vicki is an active member of the Academy of Nutrition and Dietetics, having served as Chair of the Nutrition Entrepreneurs Dietetic Practice Group (DPG), newsletter editor of the Food and Culinary Professionals DPG, and Chair of the Member Services Advisory Committee.

Vicki lives to eat well with her husband, two active youngsters, and their precocious pet pug. With a passion for cultivating healthy lifestyles simply, one craving at a time, Vicki created her recipe and lifestyle blog, www. simplecravingsrealfood.com. Join her there in your kitchen today!

The Academy of Nutrition and Dietetics was founded in Cleveland, Ohio, in 1917, by a visionary group of women dedicated to helping the government conserve food and improve the public's health and nutrition during World War I. Today, the Academy of Nutrition and Dietetics is the world's largest organization of food and nutrition professionals with more than 75,000 members committed to improving health and advancing the profession of dietetics through research, education, and advocacy.

Members of the Academy include registered dietitian nutritionists (RDN); nutrition and dietetic technicians, registered (NDTR); other dietetics professionals holding undergraduate and advanced degrees in nutrition and dietetics; and students. Dietetics practitioners work in healthcare systems, home healthcare, foodservice, business, and research and educational organizations, as well as in private practice. As vital members of medical teams in hospitals, long-term-care facilities, and health maintenance organizations, they provide medical nutrition therapy — using specific nutrition services to treat chronic conditions, illnesses, or injuries. Community-based dietetics practitioners provide health promotion, disease prevention, and wellness services.

Learn more at www.eatright.org.

Dedication

I dedicate this book, first and foremost, to my children, Grant and Samantha, whose precious tummies and minds I try to feed well every day. You make living fun! Plus, my husband, Scott, who offers me worlds of wisdom, encouragement, and a daily dose of sweet reality. You are always in my heart.

I also dedicate this book to the numerous real people I've had the pleasure of meeting who struggle with making lasting lifestyle changes. You are not alone. "Take it one moment at a time" is — and always will be — my motto!

Author's Acknowledgments

As I reflect on the process of writing this book — from the late nights and early mornings to the copious notes, edits, and questions that writing conjures up — it is here that I can sit back and say, "thank you." First, I want to offer my sincerest gratitude to my family — writing a book involves the whole household (even our "cat-dog," Stella). Plus, my dear friends who continue to push me forward — even going so far as to plan yoga retreats, in the name of research for this book! You are the best, Kristen Avini. Thank you, Mom, for always giving me something to laugh about and fostering my passion to follow my dreams. I appreciate that we were all in this together.

I want to thank everyone who touched this project at the Academy of Nutrition and Dietetics for offering editorial magic to promotional input, as well as continued energy to see this book come to fruition. It's been a collective labor of love. Thank you to my acquisitions editor, Tracy Boggier, and my project editor, Elizabeth Kuball, for knowing when to crack the whip. I can appreciate it now! Plus, Jamie Shifley, MS, RDN, LDN, director of the coordinated nutrition program at the University of Illinois at Chicago, for her support in the classroom for this project. Many thanks to graduate student and dietetic intern, Faith Moores, for contributing some creative recipes to this book. The support, guidance, and cooperation I got along the way has truly been heart-warming.

Last, but not least, to the professional community around me. I am in awe of the bounty of resources, friendships, and guidance that I've been privy to over my 15 years as a registered dietitian nutritionist. The positive energy is contagious and it continues to inspire my career in infinite ways.

Publisher's Acknowledgments

Senior Acquisitions Editor: Tracy Boggier

Project Editor: Elizabeth Kuball

Copy Editor: Elizabeth Kuball

Technical Editor: Rachel Nix, RDN

Production Editor: Kumar Chellappan

Nutrition Analyst: Rachel Nix, RDN

Recipe Tester: Emily Nolan

Cover Image: Syda Productions/Shutterstock

Apple & Mac

iPad For Dummies,
6th Edition
978-1-118-72306-7

iPhone For Dummies,
7th Edition
978-1-118-69083-3

Macs All-in-One
For Dummies, 4th Edition
978-1-118-82210-4

OS X Mavericks
For Dummies
978-1-118-69188-5

Blogging & Social Media

Facebook For Dummies,
5th Edition
978-1-118-63312-0

Social Media Engagement
For Dummies
978-1-118-53019-1

WordPress For Dummies,
6th Edition
978-1-118-79161-5

Business

Stock Investing
For Dummies, 4th Edition
978-1-118-37678-2

Investing For Dummies,
6th Edition
978-0-470-90545-6

Personal Finance
For Dummies, 7th Edition
978-1-118-11785-9

QuickBooks 2014
For Dummies
978-1-118-72005-9

Small Business Marketing
Kit For Dummies,
3rd Edition
978-1-118-31183-7

Careers

Job Interviews
For Dummies, 4th Edition
978-1-118-11290-8

Job Searching with Social
Media For Dummies,
2nd Edition
978-1-118-67856-5

Personal Branding
For Dummies
978-1-118-11792-7

Resumes For Dummies,
6th Edition
978-0-470-87361-8

Starting an Etsy Business
For Dummies, 2nd Edition
978-1-118-59024-9

Diet & Nutrition

Belly Fat Diet For Dummies
978-1-118-34585-6

Mediterranean Diet
For Dummies
978-1-118-71525-3

Nutrition For Dummies,
5th Edition
978-0-470-93231-5

Digital Photography

Digital SLR Photography
All-in-One For Dummies,
2nd Edition
978-1-118-59082-9

Digital SLR Video &
Filmmaking For Dummies
978-1-118-36598-4

Photoshop Elements 12
For Dummies
978-1-118-72714-0

Gardening

Herb Gardening
For Dummies, 2nd Edition
978-0-470-61778-6

Gardening with Free-Range
Chickens For Dummies
978-1-118-54754-0

Health

Boosting Your Immunity
For Dummies
978-1-118-40200-9

Diabetes For Dummies,
4th Edition
978-1-118-29447-5

Living Paleo For Dummies
978-1-118-29405-5

Big Data

Big Data For Dummies
978-1-118-50422-2

Data Visualization
For Dummies
978-1-118-50289-1

Hadoop For Dummies
978-1-118-60755-8

Language &
Foreign Language

500 Spanish Verbs
For Dummies
978-1-118-02382-2

English Grammar
For Dummies, 2nd Edition
978-0-470-54664-2

French All-in-One
For Dummies
978-1-118-22815-9

German Essentials
For Dummies
978-1-118-18422-6

Italian For Dummies,
2nd Edition
978-1-118-00465-4

Available in print and e-book formats.

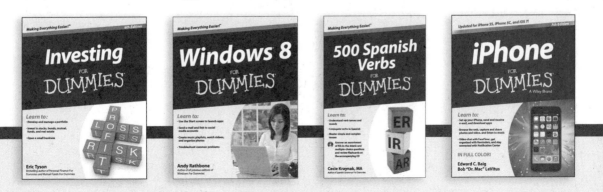

Available wherever books are sold. **For more information or to order direct visit www.dummies.com**

Math & Science

Algebra I For Dummies,
2nd Edition
978-0-470-55964-2

Anatomy and Physiology
For Dummies, 2nd Edition
978-0-470-92326-9

Astronomy For Dummies,
3rd Edition
978-1-118-37697-3

Biology For Dummies,
2nd Edition
978-0-470-59875-7

Chemistry For Dummies,
2nd Edition
978-1-118-00730-3

1001 Algebra II Practice
Problems For Dummies
978-1-118-44662-1

Microsoft Office

Excel 2013 For Dummies
978-1-118-51012-4

Office 2013 All-in-One
For Dummies
978-1-118-51636-2

PowerPoint 2013
For Dummies
978-1-118-50253-2

Word 2013 For Dummies
978-1-118-49123-2

Music

Blues Harmonica
For Dummies
978-1-118-25269-7

Guitar For Dummies,
3rd Edition
978-1-118-11554-1

iPod & iTunes
For Dummies, 10th Edition
978-1-118-50864-0

Programming

Beginning Programming
with C For Dummies
978-1-118-73763-7

Excel VBA Programming
For Dummies, 3rd Edition
978-1-118-49037-2

Java For Dummies,
6th Edition
978-1-118-40780-6

Religion & Inspiration

The Bible For Dummies
978-0-7645-5296-0

Buddhism For Dummies,
2nd Edition
978-1-118-02379-2

Catholicism For Dummies,
2nd Edition
978-1-118-07778-8

Self-Help & Relationships

Beating Sugar Addiction
For Dummies
978-1-118-54645-1

Meditation For Dummies,
3rd Edition
978-1-118-29144-3

Seniors

Laptops For Seniors
For Dummies, 3rd Edition
978-1-118-71105-7

Computers For Seniors
For Dummies, 3rd Edition
978-1-118-11553-4

iPad For Seniors
For Dummies, 6th Edition
978-1-118-72826-0

Social Security
For Dummies
978-1-118-20573-0

Smartphones & Tablets

Android Phones
For Dummies, 2nd Edition
978-1-118-72030-1

Nexus Tablets
For Dummies
978-1-118-77243-0

Samsung Galaxy S 4
For Dummies
978-1-118-64222-1

Samsung Galaxy Tabs
For Dummies
978-1-118-77294-2

Test Prep

ACT For Dummies,
5th Edition
978-1-118-01259-8

ASVAB For Dummies,
3rd Edition
978-0-470-63760-9

GRE For Dummies,
7th Edition
978-0-470-88921-3

Officer Candidate Tests
For Dummies
978-0-470-59876-4

Physician's Assistant Exam
For Dummies
978-1-118-11556-5

Series 7 Exam For Dummies
978-0-470-09932-2

Windows 8

Windows 8.1 All-in-One
For Dummies
978-1-118-82087-2

Windows 8.1 For Dummies
978-1-118-82121-3

Windows 8.1 For Dummies,
Book + DVD Bundle
978-1-118-82107-7

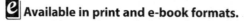

Available in print and e-book formats.

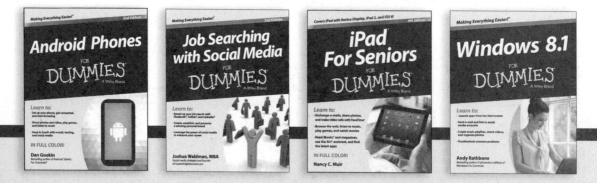

Available wherever books are sold. **For more information or to order direct visit www.dummies.com**

Take Dummies with you everywhere you go!

Whether you are excited about e-books, want more from the web, must have your mobile apps, or are swept up in social media, Dummies makes everything easier.

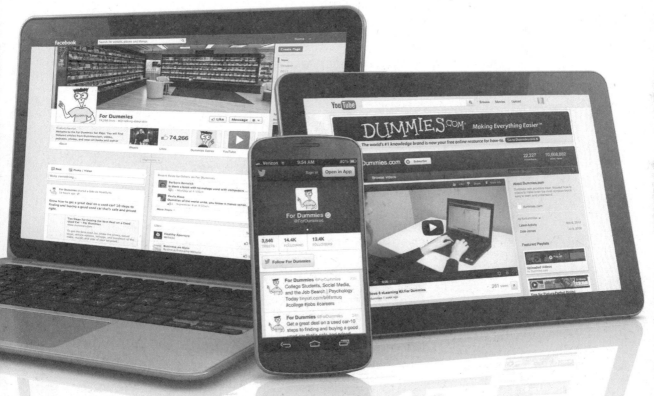

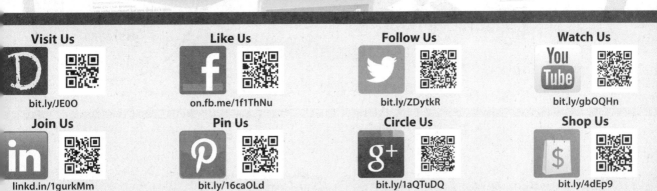

For Dummies is the global leader in the reference category and one of the most trusted and highly regarded brands in the world. No longer just focused on books, customers now have access to the For Dummies content they need in the format they want. Let us help you develop a solution that will fit your brand and help you connect with your customers.

Advertising & Sponsorships

Connect with an engaged audience on a powerful multimedia site, and position your message alongside expert how-to content.

Targeted ads • Video • Email marketing • Microsites • Sweepstakes sponsorship

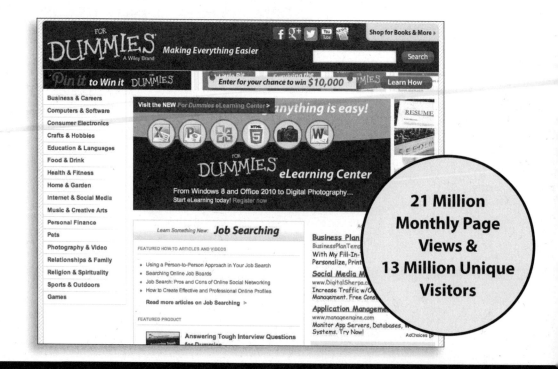

21 Million Monthly Page Views & 13 Million Unique Visitors